COMMISSIONING
HEALTH +
WELLBEING

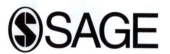

COMMISSIONING
HEALTH +
WELLBEING

CHRIS HEGINBOTHAM
KAREN NEWBIGGING

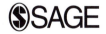

Los Angeles | London | New Delhi
Singapore | Washington DC

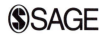

Los Angeles | London | New Delhi
Singapore | Washington DC

SAGE Publications Ltd
1 Oliver's Yard
55 City Road
London EC1Y 1SP

SAGE Publications Inc.
2455 Teller Road
Thousand Oaks, California 91320

SAGE Publications India Pvt Ltd
B 1/I 1 Mohan Cooperative Industrial Area
Mathura Road
New Delhi 110 044

SAGE Publications Asia-Pacific Pte Ltd
3 Church Street
#10-04 Samsung Hub
Singapore 049483

Editor: Alex Clabburn
Assistant editor: Emma Milman
Production editor: Katie Forsythe
Copyeditor: Gemma Marren
Proofreader: Anna Gilding
Marketing manager: Tamara Navaratnam
Cover design: Wendy Scott
Typeset by: C&M Digitals (P) Ltd, Chennai, India
Printed in Great Britain by Henry Ling Limited, at
the Dorset Press, Dorchester, DT1 1HD

Library of Congress Control Number: 2013934400

British Library Cataloguing in Publication data

A catalogue record for this book is available from
the British Library

MIX
Paper from
responsible sources

FSC
www.fsc.org   **FSC® C013985**

ISBN 978-1-4462-5254-3
ISBN 978-1-4462-5255-0 (pbk)

For Emily, Sarah, Laura, Elizabeth, Ewan and Amber, and future generations.

Contents

List of Figures and Tables

About the Authors

Prof Chris Heginbotham is Emeritus Professor of Mental Health Policy and Management at the University of Central Lancashire, holds an honorary chair in the Institute of Clinical Education at the Medical School, Warwick University, and a Visiting Professorship at the University of Cumbria. He was National Director of Mind for much of the 1980s, when he represented the World Federation for Mental Health at the UN Commission on Human Rights in Geneva; and he has held a number of Chief Executive positions in the NHS, including Chief Executive at different times of two health authorities and two NHS Trusts. His most recent post prior to joining the University of Central Lancashire was as Chief Executive of the Mental Health Act Commission. In the 1980s and early 1990s Chris held non-executive positions with various health authorities. He is presently a non-executive director of the Lancashire Care NHS Foundation Trust and a Board member of the Global Health Equity Foundation, Geneva, where he leads on health equity research.

Dr Karen Newbigging qualified as a clinical psychologist in 1981 and is a Chartered Psychologist and has experience of commissioning mental health services. Since 1999, Karen has been involved in research, consultancy and organisational development and worked with a broad range of organisations on mental health system development and action to tackle inequalities, including co-leading a national programme on gender inequalities and mental health. Karen is currently Senior Lecturer in the Health Services Management Centre at the University of Birmingham and undertakes research on mental wellbeing as well as contributing to postgraduate programmes for commissioners on health and wellbeing. With Chris Heginbotham, Karen co-authored a toolkit and leadership briefing for commissioners on commissioning for mental health and wellbeing.

Acknowledgements

This book arose from a research and development project funded initially by the National Mental Health Development Unit of the Department of Health between 2008 and 2010. We are grateful to Jonathan Campion, Gregor Henderson, Kate O'Hara and Jude Stansfield especially for their help and support in preparing the booklets resulting from that project on which this book is partially based. Those booklets, the executive briefing, *Commissioning Mental Wellbeing* (Heginbotham and Newbigging, 2010) and the fuller guidance, *Commissioning Mental Wellbeing for All* (Newbigging and Heginbotham, 2010) were published by the University of Central Lancashire (UCLan) where Chris Heginbotham is now an Emeritus Professor and Karen Newbigging works as a Principal Lecturer. We would like to thank colleagues at UCLan and the project steering group for their support for the earlier booklets, who in addition to those already cited include Andy Bennett, Sarah Carter, Michael Clark, Keith Foster, Louise Howell, Martin Seymour, Elizabeth Wade. We are indebted to Margaret Barry, Lynne Friedli, Martin Knapp, David McDaid and Michael Parsonage, and many researchers too numerous to mention for discussions on health and wellbeing opportunities and especially the results of economic analyses. Many people were consulted in the preparation of the book, including health and social care commissioners and public health professionals.

We are grateful to the World Health Organization especially, for permission to reproduce Figures 3.2, 3.7 and 3.8, and to EuroHealthNet, particularly Clive Needle and Caroline Costongs, for permission to reproduce Figures 3.3 and 3.4, and to all those in the following listing for permission to reproduce diagrams, graphs and tables. It goes without saying, but we will say it anyway, that all omissions and any mistakes, which we hope are very few, remain our responsibility.

Staff at Sage have been nothing but helpful throughout production of the book. In particular, we would like to thank Emma Milman and Katie Forsythe for working with us tirelessly and patiently in dealing with queries and ensuring that all the referencing was accurate. Any final imperfections, of course, remain fully our responsibility.

Publisher's
Acknowledgements

Churchill Livingstone (Margaret Barry and Rachel Jenkins) for Figure 1.1: Opportunities for mental health promotion: a population perspective (adapted from Barry and Jenkins, 2007).

World Health Organization (WHO) for 'A systemic representation of social determinants of health' adapted from Solar and Irwin (2007) and the report of the WHO/Commission on the Social Determinants of Health (2008), used in Figure 3.2.

EuroHealthNet (Clive Needle, Ingrid Stegeman and Caroline Costongs) for the example in Figures 3.3 and 3.4 of socio-economic gradient in Ireland showing life expectancy by social class (taken from Stegeman and Costongs, 2012: 25) and subjective general health in one parent and two parent families (Stegeman and Costongs, 2012: 67).

Dr Somen Banerjee, Associate Director of Public Health, NHS Tower Hamlets (15 July 2010) for histograms used in Figure 3.5, showing mortality from all circulatory diseases (selected local government areas) showing the twofold difference between boroughs, and Figure 3.6, showing differential mortality for CHD and diabetes, with figures for the national picture, London and three London boroughs.

World Health Organization (WHO) for permission to reproduce diagrams in Figure 3.7, related to the Urban HEART process and the simplified diagram in Figure 3.8, explaining the way that Urban HEART is used, as redrawn by the authors from the source of the basic table: Urban HEART, www.who.int/kobe_centre/measuring/urbanheart/en/.

Longevity Science Advisory Panel 2011 for Figures 6.1 and 6.2 based on 'Life expectancy: past and future variations by socioeconomic group in England and Wales' (www.longevitypanel.co.uk), which was adapted from Tables 1b (males) and 4b (females), Life expectancy by NS-SEC class, males/females at age 65, *Statistical Bulletin: Trends in life expectancy by the National Statistics, Socio-economic Classification 1982–2006*, 22 February 2011. Office for National Statistics, 2011: 6 (www.ons.gov.uk/ons/rel/hsq/health-statisticsquarterly/trends-in-life-expectancy-by-the-national-statistics-socio-economicclassification-1982-2006/index.html) © Crown Copyright 2011. This information is licensed under the terms of the Open Government License v1.0 (www.nationalarchives.gov.uk/doc/open-government-licence/open-government-licence.htm).

Health and Safety Executive for Figure 7.2, Number and rate of fatal injury to workers, 1992/93–2011/12. Source: www.hse.gov.uk/statistics/fatals.htm (accessed on 25 July 2012).

Health and Safety Executive for Figure 7.3, Total number of cases (prevalence) of workplace stress has continued to rise and new cases (incidence) of work-related stress in GB 2001/02–2010/11 Source: www.hse.gov.uk/statistics/causdis/stress/index.htm (accessed on 25 July 2012).

Dr Shahrad Taheri, University of Birmingham, for permission to use the diagram at Figure 8.1 from a presentation given on 20 October 2012.

Royal College of Psychiatrists for permission to use two graphs at Figure 9.1 from a paper by Weich et al. (2012).

Health Promoting School image from the Australian Women and Children's Health Network, Centre for Health Promotion, for Figure 6.4. Reproduced by kind permission of the Centre for Health Promotion.

National Implementation Research Network at the Louis de la Parte Florida Mental Health Institute, University of South Florida, for Figure 10.1. Implementing evidence-based programmes: a two-step process. Adapted from Fixsen et al. (2005).

Abbreviations

CBT	cognitive behavioural therapy
CCG(s)	Clinical Commissioning Group(s)
CHD	coronary heart disease
COPD	Chronic obstructive pulmonary disease
CSDH	Commission on the Social Determinants of Health
CVD	cerebrovascular disease
DH	Department of Health
EGA	Equity Gap Analysis
GWAS	Genome Wide Association Studies
HPS	Health Promoting School
HWB(s)	Health and Wellbeing Board(s)
IPV	Intimate partner violence
JHWS	Joint Health and Wellbeing Strategies
JSNA	joint strategic needs assessments
LA	Local Authority
LOAD	late onset Alzheimer's disease
MCI	mild cognitive impairment
MWIA	Mental Wellbeing Impact Assessment
NCB	NHS Commissioning Board
nef	New Economics Foundation
NICE	National Institute for Health and Clinical Excellence
ONS	Office for National Statistics
PCT	Primary Care Trust
PD	Parkinson's disease
PPD	postpartum depression
PPW	positive psychological wellbeing
SCIE	Social Care Institute for Excellence
SEL	social and emotional learning
SNP	single nucleotide polymorphisms
WEMWBS	Warwick Edinburgh Mental Wellbeing Scale

CHAPTER 1

Introduction

Health and wellbeing are elusive concepts and the aim of this book is to support commissioners translate current aspirations of public mental health into tangible commissioning strategies. This book provides a carefully structured and comprehensive look at the resources designed to improve population health and wellbeing outcomes. It is being published at a time when there are major changes in commissioning arrangements in England and we hope that our contribution will enable a debate within Clinical Commissioning Groups (CCGs) and Health and Wellbeing Boards (HWBs) and other emerging organisations about the possibilities for using current resources, both human and financial, by focusing on health and wellbeing as well as illness.

This chapter starts by setting the background and explains our view about positive mental health and wellbeing, making the general case for investments by health and social care commissioners in wellbeing interventions.

1.1 Introduction

The importance of mental and physical wellbeing and the positive benefits it brings to individuals and communities is now widely recognised. These include better health and health-related behaviours, greater resilience, an enhanced capacity for creativity and innovation, stronger social networks, positive relationships and connected communities as well as reduced mortality (Aked et al, 2010; DH, 2009a; National Mental Wellbeing Impact Assessment (MWIA) Collaborative, 2011). In the last six years, there have been several valuable reports published by the New Economics Foundation (nef) (see, for example, *Measuring Wellbeing in Policy*, 2008; *Five Ways to Wellbeing: The Evidence*, 2008),[1] the Government Office for Science (the Foresight Report, 2008) and the Marmot Review in 2010 (Marmot, 2010). The National Institute for Health and Clinical Excellence (NICE) and the Department of Health (DH) have also published a range of reports, summarising the evidence base and promoting commissioning for mental wellbeing as a key strategic programme. Together these reports provide an evidence base for why it makes sense to focus on wellbeing and the role played by the social determinants of health, and a bibliography is available as an Appendix. The reason wellbeing has gained so much attention is the understanding that mental capital is needed to enable us to adapt to the challenges ahead, particularly to those of the global economic recession, climate change and its consequences, population growth and its effect in a reduction of resources, and greater equality between nations and continents. Even at times of austerity, an emphasis on social protection and active labour market programmes that support personal development, as well as simply getting people into a job, can encourage and promote wellbeing.

Wellbeing has become a more accepted way of understanding how people feel about the society in which they live. Since November 2010, when the Office for National Statistics (ONS) launched the Measuring National Well-being programme, a set of measures has been available that complements figures for Gross Domestic Product (GDP), offer a greater understanding of the way people feel about changes taking place in society and assist ordinary people to understand what is important to the country (ONS, 2010). Bhutan was perhaps the first country actively to consider a Gross National Happiness (GNH) quotient, but the UK may soon be catching up.[2]

Before we go any further, however, we need to explore what we mean by wellbeing. Although physical and mental wellbeing are inextricably linked, our focus is on mental wellbeing. Mental wellbeing is a multi-dimensional concept and is the foundation for positive health and effective functioning for an individual and for a community. We explore the concept of mental wellbeing in more detail in Chapter 2; however, the terminology is problematic and work in Scotland has found it can evoke strong emotions. There is a paradox. If we speak about 'health' alone, it will not be clear that we mean the totality of health-promoting psychological and physical interventions that have wellbeing as the goal; if we speak about 'mental health', it will not be clear that we mean comprehensive positive mental health as well as preventive strategies to reduce the risk and incidence of mental illness. We are rightly concerned with achieving positive mental health as a concomitant of a wider description of wellbeing; improvements to mental wellbeing come from improvements in physical health, and in this way physical and mental health are intimately connected. The term 'mental health' often, indeed usually, conjures up in the reader's mind the idea of mental health *care*, or in other words mental illness services. In the discussion here we do not want to place any more than marginal emphasis on mental illness or services labelled as mental health care; our purpose is the positive mental health that stems from those aspects of society that support flourishing and resilience (see Chapter 2) whether those are social, familial, psychological, biological, organisational, economic or political determinants of wellbeing. Consequently we have called the book *Commissioning Health and Wellbeing*, not *Mental* Health and Wellbeing, hopefully for what are now obvious reasons.

In this book, we want to offer ideas that will enable commissioners to commission to achieve physical and mental health wellbeing. First, the focus will be on public (mental) health in addition to primary, secondary and tertiary prevention of any disease or distress where its course can be modified by early preventive interventions that reduce or ameliorate distress such that the long-term consequences are much improved. Second, we are concerned with cost-effective interventions in health and social care that support or improve wellbeing, for individuals, their families and communities. Third, we are concerned with the health and wellbeing of specific populations whose situation and social processes further disadvantage them and increase their vulnerability to poor health. Inevitably this includes people with a diagnosis of mental illness and so we are also concerned with interventions that will assist with recovery of service users towards the objectives they set themselves for their lives. We are not concerned with mental health care (mental illness services) except where these impinge on the generic promotion and prevention agenda; but we are interested in commissioning health and social care that promotes wellbeing, applying lessons from the literature wisely and correctly to achieve savings and longer-term benefits for wider society.

1.2 Improving health and wellbeing

Mental health as a positive concept is a key element of what we mean by health and wellbeing. Perhaps mental wellbeing might be a better term. Wellbeing is a broad construct that encompasses a variety of theoretical approaches including eudai-monic wellbeing, hedonic wellbeing, and social wellbeing (Gallagher et al., 2009). Whatever term we use though, mental health is an essential component of general health. In other words there is no health without mental health (Royal College of Psychiatrists, 2010). Mental wellbeing is a critical asset in the fight for improved health – it is both an objective and a support on the road to that objective. This means it is a resource both at an individual level, enabling people to cope with the demands of everyday living and the unexpected – in other words it is concerned with resilience – and at a social level, fostering stronger and sustainable social rela-tionships and communities. It is a resource for the long-term social and economic prosperity of society.

In contrast to psychological 'ill-being' (i.e. pervasive negative feelings and poor func-tioning in life), positive psychological wellbeing (PPW) reflects the positive components of psychological health that characterise individuals who feel good about life and func-tion well (Keyes and Annas, 2009; in contrast to Kashdan et al., 2008 with whom this paper disagrees. See also Tiberius and Plakias, 2010). Improving mental wellbeing requires efforts to be focused on promoting wellbeing for communities and individuals and on those at risk of poor mental health: communities, social networks and the envi-ronment play a central role alongside education, transport, health and social services, employment, financial security and leisure opportunities in strengthening resilience both at an individual and a community level. Responsibility for promoting mental wellbeing extends across all disciplines and government departments and encompasses a concern for social values, culture, economic and social, as well as health policies. It includes approaches that involve and strengthen the active participation of local communities and local people, particularly those from vulnerable groups, who are central to improving mental wellbeing. Consequently, commissioning for mental wellbeing should be focused on delivering the best possible health and wellbeing outcomes through the best use of the available information and resources.

Commissioning for mental wellbeing involves considering three sets of objectives: health and wellbeing promotion for the whole population; primary, secondary and tertiary prevention of potential health and social risks; and wellbeing developments for those living with or recovering from mental illness. The Figure 1.1 summarises this approach and provides a useful framework for developing a strategic approach to com-missioning for mental wellbeing. The first three columns are the focus for this book – positive wellbeing for all; prevention; and promoting health for those with incipient or actual mental health problems – but the last column is not within the remit of the book as that describes mental health services. However, this is an important area for commis-sioners, who will be concerned to commission mental health services that promote recovery and wellbeing.

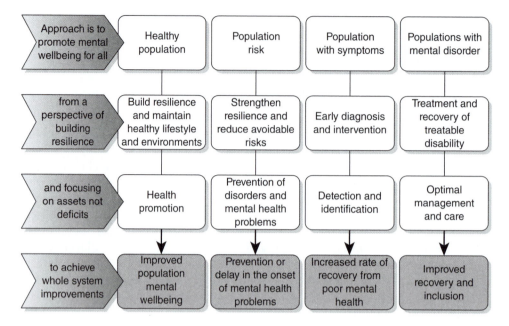

Figure 1.1 Opportunities for mental health promotion: a population perspective (adapted from Barry and Jenkins, 2007)

1.3 Commissioning for outcomes

At a time of austerity it may seem naïve, even foolish, to suggest health promoting and preventive interventions; yet there is a strong case to be made on the basis of the evidence available for a range of outcomes including social and economic ones. Improving population mental wellbeing has the potential to contribute to far-reaching improvements in physical and mental health, a better quality of life, higher educational attainment, economic wellbeing and reduction in crime and anti-social behaviour. The main outcomes, which have been well evidenced, are illustrated in Box 1.1 (see, for example, Kim-Cohen et al., 2003; Saxena et al., 2006; Barry and Jenkins, 2007; Friedli and Parsonage, 2007).

The foundations for positive mental wellbeing are laid down in early life and as we grow and mature through our teenage years. This is when we learn most rapidly. The quality of the relationships and experiences we have in our early years and the learning that we do about our emotions and our relationships as we grow up are vital. For example, half of lifetime mental illness (excluding dementia) is already present by the age of 14 (Kessler et al., 2005) so the early years provide a critical opportunity for intervention. Mental wellbeing is important across the life span and the health and wellbeing of older generations affects that of younger people. Thus, better outcomes are likely to be achieved through the adoption of a life course approach that recognises that mental capital, as discussed in Chapter 2, is a resource we develop and use throughout our life and is available to and built by others, reflecting our interdependencies and interconnectedness.

> ## Box 1.1 Advantages and outcomes of focusing on health and wellbeing
>
> - Increased quality of life and overall wellbeing.
>
> - Increased life expectancy, provide protection from coronary heart disease, improve health outcomes from a range of long-term conditions (e.g. diabetes).
>
> - Reduce risks to health through influencing positive health behaviours, such as reductions in alcohol and substance use.
>
> - Reduced health inequalities – both physical and mental health – and impact positively on the social determinants of health.
>
> - Improved educational attainment, outcomes and subsequent occupation.
>
> - Safer communities with less crime.
>
> - Improved productivity and employment retention, reduced sickness absence from work and reduced 'presenteeism'.
>
> - Reduced levels of poor mental health and mental illness and the adverse consequences of mental illness or distress (NB wellbeing is *not* the opposite of mental illness).

1.4 The case for commissioning for mental wellbeing

Current health (NHS) and local authorities' policy is that commissioning for health, wellbeing and independence[3] is as important as commissioning for 'illness' (see, for example, North Yorkshire County Council, 2007; Bennett et al., 2011; DH, 2011a). This emphasis includes a growing awareness of the negative impact of poor mental wellbeing and indeed poor mental health, as well as opportunities for intervention at a population and individual level. The case for mental wellbeing improvement is an increased quality of life and overall wellbeing, and wider health benefits to individuals and the population. Mental wellbeing is entwined with physical health with the potential for positive feedback both ways.

There are five arguments that support the case for commissioning for health and wellbeing: demographic changes; an increasingly robust evidence base; the economic dimension – invest to prevent and save; tackling social injustice and promoting equalities; and underpinning all of these, a moral argument. Readers will have their own preferences but we take the approach that together they make a strong case for commissioning for wellbeing and that not to do so wholeheartedly is merely a shift in lexicon rather than the paradigm change that is needed. We will explore these arguments in this book but want to introduce them here to provide a starting point for the subsequent material.

a) Demographic changes

Demographic changes over the forthcoming decades will place very significant pressures on individuals, communities, local authorities and health agencies. This will be especially true of the growing numbers of older people, one fifth of whom over the age of 80 will have dementia and another fifth will be unable to carry out the usual activities of daily living. A substantial number, perhaps 10%, will have diabetes or at least one other long-term condition, such as cerebrovascular disease (CVD), heart failure, end stage renal failure associated with hypertension, and possibly digestive tract disorders. This will have far-reaching impacts on individuals' quality of life and the budgets of statutory authorities, which are unlikely to be able to cope without a radical rethink of how we commission for a healthy older age, making investment in this area essential. In Chapter 8, we explore the interconnection between depression, diabetes and dementia as an exemplar of the inter-relationship between mental wellbeing and physical health and how wellbeing interventions for one may have a wider value. Chapter 9 considers the opportunities and assets that older people represent and how their continued contribution has both individual and social benefits.

b) An increasingly robust evidence base

The evidence for the effectiveness of wellbeing interventions has become more persuasive steadily over the preceding ten years. Gone are the days – or so they should be – when health commissioners could simply refuse to listen. Many of the health promotion objectives can be delivered through health and wellbeing interventions that are (a) much cheaper, and (b) prevent, in many cases, precisely the illnesses (or at least the worst aspect of those illnesses) that cost the NHS so much money. We recognise that this sounds like the worst sort of rhetoric; but we would ask anyone reading the book to do so with an open mind and reflect on the quantity and quality of the evidence. Of course not everything is as well evidenced as the best, but that is true of much acute medical and surgical care now. Chapters 6 to 9 provide an overview of the evidence for significant interventions for children, young people and adults, including older adults. This is a partial look at the evidence but the areas we have chosen we think represent the key areas for commissioners to consider, as a starting point to improving population wellbeing.

c) Invest to prevent and save

Commissioning public mental health and wellbeing offers significant potential savings by strengthening protective factors and reducing risk factors, which will have significant implications for health and social care usage elsewhere in the system. Taking a life course approach, as we suggested previously, places a premium on early intervention, but there are many interventions that are available for older adults. As our wider preventive strategy develops it must be hoped that disability and death will be pushed away and the life curve (quality against quantity) will be 'squared-off', as shown in Figure 1.2.

Public health has an important role in identifying locally the opportunities for investment in wellbeing that will have an impact elsewhere in the system. Lower health

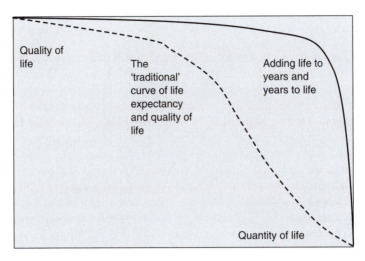

Quality of life

The 'traditional' curve of life expectancy and quality of life

Adding life to years and years to life

Quantity of life

Figure 1.2 Adding years to life and (especially) life to years 'squares' the life expectancy curve

care utilisation is also likely to result so that investment in mental wellbeing interventions will have positive impacts in other parts of the health and social care system, not to mention the savings that may accrue in other sectors. Even at a time of austerity, focusing on wellbeing means that we give precedence to positive psychological health and investing in people's resilience. This places an emphasis on health promotion and illness prevention, and by preventing illness occurring, and taking a long-term perspective on such matters as child physical and sexual abuse, it will both improve wellbeing and save significant levels of financial resources for reinvestment elsewhere. It seems perverse that, just when people are losing their jobs as a result of the recession, the government should reduce the benefits that have been part of the social contract, offering social protection that has sustained individuals and families, reduced their anxiety and made it easier for them to find employment again. Some of those savings become available quite quickly, within two years; some are only realised after longish periods of time, over 20 or more years. Some of the savings are not in health or social care but appear in other areas of the public sector: criminal justice, the prison service, education, housing and so on. However, heartening news from the Spearhead[4] group of local authorities is that a programme to tackle inequalities that was begun in the early to mid 'naughties' is now bearing fruit, after ten years or so.

Certain interventions are more cost-effective than others, certain interventions are easier to implement. We will see as we explore different areas for interventions, some objectives will be more achievable than others. What we have described above is summarised in Figure 1.3. This suggests a more holistic reality in which it can be seen that the three areas are not mutually exclusive. They overlap in ways that are frequently demonstrated by the outcome achieved in an area that differs from the one in which the intervention is targeted.

Positive health messages are relevant to people with mental illness as much as anyone else; wellbeing for people with mental illness is one of the elements of a proportionate approach that focuses on those deemed at risk; and universal preventive strategies can bring benefits in positive health and wellbeing in addition to the specific outcomes to be achieved by the intervention.

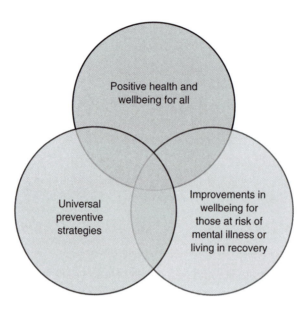

Figure 1.3 The inter-relationship of the three aspects of health and wellbeing

d) Social justice and promoting equalities

One of the most important arguments supporting a focus on public mental health is the value of social justice in promoting equity and equality. Prevention and health promotion are two of the most significant aspects of health and social care. Why is it so difficult for politicians to recognise the value of prevention instead of treatment? This is especially true in relation to mental health. Mental health, and by that we mean positive mental health for all, is the other side of the coin of social justice. Being mentally healthy means that our basic needs have been met and we have been accorded autonomy, resources, and acceptance. For example, it is immensely difficult to get people to become engaged in the higher order features of their lives (e.g. as described by Maslow's hierarchy of needs – see Figure 1.4) if their more basic needs are not being met or are likely not to be met.

The Secretary of State for Health, the NHS Commissioning Board (NCB) and Clinical Commissioning Groups have legal duties under the Health and Social Care Act 2012 (HM Government, 2012) in relation to reducing health inequalities. In Chapter 3 we consider equity in health and social care and recognise the value of the social determinants of health. By focusing on food, road transport and air pollution, global warming, decent housing and so on we will prevent many of the deprivation-borne disorders from forming. In Chapter 6 we demonstrate how poor parenting leads to poor child rearing, perhaps as a result of alcohol-driven intimate partner violence, and will almost certainly mean a life of lower opportunity and poorer achievement. But it doesn't have to be like that. By making social justice our aim we can ensure that everyone's life is improved; and incidentally we ensure as well that the resources are spread between people in spaces of deprivation (Popay, 2012) rather than being spent sometimes in too bureaucratic a manner by well-heeled professional staff.

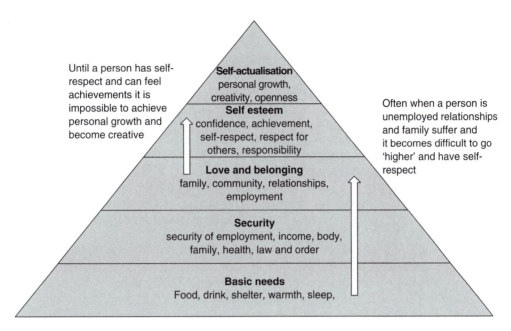

Until a person has self-respect and can feel achievements it is impossible to achieve personal growth and become creative

Self-actualisation
personal growth,
creativity, openness

Self esteem
confidence, achievement,
self-respect, respect for
others, responsibility

Love and belonging
family, community, relationships,
employment

Security
security of employment, income, body,
family, health, law and order

Basic needs
Food, drink, shelter, warmth, sleep,

Often when a person is unemployed relationships and family suffer and it becomes difficult to go 'higher' and have self-respect

Figure 1.4 Maslow's hierarchy of need (redrawn by the authors from Maslow, 1943)

e) The moral argument

Health promotion, illness prevention and wellbeing generation should draw on evidence and ethics as two related systems of reasoning. At the same time values (of individuals, groups, communities and the general population) are a crucial aspect in taking a 'full-field' standpoint (see Fulford et al., 2012; Heginbotham, 2012). The evidence and values should be made explicit as should the ethical basis of the way health promotion and prevention are implemented (Carter et al., 2011). Amartya Sen (2002), for example, advocates capabilities as an alternative to a utilitarian approach to welfare, opening up opportunities; recasting disability as '*capabilities deprivation because it interferes with a person's ability to make valued choices and participate fully in society*' (Hopper, 2007: 874). Much commissioning is currently based on a deficit model and we explore the implications for an assets-based approach for transformational change below. Commissioning is thus a moral endeavour, with assumptions about humanity constructed and reproduced through our policies and commissioning intentions.

1.5 Improving mental wellbeing

Critical decisions will need to be made about ways of focusing effort in those areas which are most likely to reap benefits. Clear direction will be required concerning where resources should be invested and focusing efforts on initiatives that are known to be effective and have been tried and tested. This does not mean stifling local innovation but rather balancing creative local practice with a commitment to implementing and scaling up evidence-based programmes that have been clearly shown to have worked across different settings. For example, there is a very robust evidence base concerning the effectiveness of interventions in the early years with families and young children. We will see in Chapter 6 how early years interventions and parenting skills can improve life chances, and in Chapter 8 how, if those interventions were applied, they could help to improve diabetes self-management.

The assets approach to health offers the opportunity for citizens to take control of their lives and to access a range of assets in doing so. The deficits model considers illness and death as inevitable and defines a pathway as shown on the left of Figure 1.5. Conversely the assets model recognises the value of personal control and that the use of assets in the community (or social environment in which the person lives) can help to identify disease earlier, reduce the need for health care resources and support recovery. In this way we can see that the deficits model and the assets model are not mutually exclusive (Pavlekovic et al., 2011).

Personal and community assets, on their own, will not resolve serious disease or offer appropriate treatments; but similarly, the deficits model on its own condemns many people, usually those living in deprived communities, to existing with curable or at least modifiable disease. By constructing disease (failure of function) or illness (failure of agency) (Fulford, 2004) in new ways, we can see what assets we need to improve function and agency; by constructing recovery as personal control over life (or treatment) objectives, it is possible to identify those aspects of the environment that will assist in achieving a healthy life.

One of the main tenets of the assets approach is to emphasise connectedness and co-production. Enabling people to connect (the first of the nef five wellbeing steps) will encourage an interest in asset finding and designation. There is in communities an 'asset unconscious', which can be found through dialogue with others. Assets 'emerge' in the interplay of language about community: often people are unaware of the physical or personal assets until they describe them during facilitated discussions. These assets have probably been there all along and simply need identification and 'permission' to be used. In Chapter 5 we consider ways of engaging communities authentically to empower local

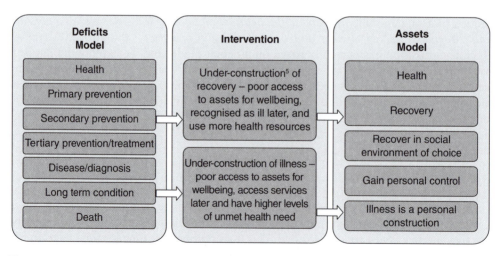

Figure 1.5 From a deficits model to an assets model

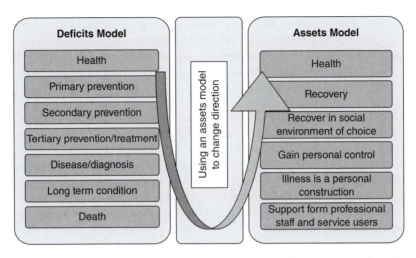

Figure 1.6 Transformative action in changing from a pathology focus to a health focus

people and to identify the assets that they have locally, which they may never have noticed, or if they did they thought would not be of value for health and wellbeing.

The model proposed above does not absolve professional or community staff – concerned with inequities in health access or disturbed by the prevalence of health inequalities borne of many years of neglect and discrimination – from tackling inequalities through determined access to the best technology and the most applicable care. The assets model does not readily achieve change for those already suffering the effects of inequity – for example, social deprivation, lack of access to health resources, early onset long-term conditions made worse by insufficient or ineffective treatments – but by developing an inclusive community-oriented assets base it will be possible to ensure an improving environment for the future. Tackling existing inequalities, however, requires some old-fashioned focus on those with disease, and the establishment of transparent targets that are used to identify the proper interventions that will bring the numbers down in line with the targets set.

1.6 Our approach

We unashamedly take a life course approach to health and wellbeing. Many of our recommendations are focused on ways in which early life experiences, both risks and protective factors, affect the health trajectory of the individual, usually adversely, later in life (see, for example, Halfon and Hochstein, 2002). In this model, health is a consequence of many factors operating through genetic, biological, behavioural, social, psychological, familial, economic and political contexts. Health adapts as the contexts in which it is 'expressed' change and develop over the life of the individual (which is one reason why wellbeing is such an intangible and slippery subject!) In this model 'health' 'takes on a trajectory that results from the cumulative influence of multiple risk and protective factors that are programmed into an individual's bio-behavioural regulatory systems during critical and sensitive time periods in development'[6] (Halfon and Hochstein, 2002). Similarly, a life course approach to the epidemiology of long-term conditions is the study of the effects on chronic disease risk of physical, mental, psychological and social exposures during pregnancy, childhood, adolescence, young adulthood and later adult life. It includes studies of 'the biological, behavioural and psychosocial pathways that operate along an individual's life course ... to influence the development of chronic diseases' (Kuh and Ben-Shlomo, 1997: 285; see also Ben-Shlomo and Kuh, 2002).

Consequently, we hope this book will help to:

- assist the development of a life course approach to health and wellbeing;
- promote those interventions that are known to work or have a good chance of providing im-provements in (mental) health and wellbeing;
- provide benefits for physical and mental health promotion and suggest preventive measures that will stop or attenuate those behaviours that lead to physical and mental problems;
- assist in building social capital within our communities;
- address inequalities in society and offer ways to address and challenge those inequalities in the way they arise and are sustained;
- achieve better outcomes for public health interventions;
- enable communities to understand and obtain improved health and social care outcomes;
- support people to take greater responsibility for improving their own health and wellbeing.

We will, in the course of the book, develop four arguments for the suggested interventions we propose. Reflecting those above, these are:

- **economics** – wellbeing makes economic sense and is cost-effective, as has been shown by nef and others;
- **equalities** – wellbeing helps to tackle health and social inequities and inequalities – it offers a vehicle for an assets-based approach to public health;
- **ethics** – promoting wellbeing through an assets-based approach (that ameliorates but does not emasculate a deficits approach) is morally the right thing to do, as is promoting the best possible psychological health available;
- **evidence** – it works where it works! (and we will try to offer the best evidence of the interventions available).

Mental wellbeing is influenced by a complex interplay of factors at an individual, social and community level (Ryan and Deci, 2001). Although wellbeing is dependent on many factors, and in an ideal world would be based on inter-sectoral and interde-partmental action across national and local government, in practice this is very diffi-cult to achieve. Place-based approaches are one way to bring resources together to focus on wellbeing and facilitate a shared vision across organisations. Whilst it is important to recognise the inter-sectoral aspects of wellbeing, there is little purpose served in idealistic pipe dreams about the best, which then becomes the enemy of the practical and achievable. We, therefore, focus unashamedly on what health and social care commissioners can do now whilst recognising and reflecting the role of other sectors, notably housing, education, transport and the role of local government, gov-ernment agencies and the third sector.

1.7 Overview of the book

Commissioning for health and wellbeing of a local population means understanding the factors that build and strengthen individual and community resilience, that enable local

communities and individuals to stay healthy, independent and interdependent and antici-
pating the risks that might jeopardise this. That requires a full understanding of local
health inequalities, their social, physical and socio-economic determinants and their implications for mental wellbeing, and finding ways to tackle those inequalities identified. Commissioning also means promoting health and social inclusion and supporting independence
through the mainstream policies and activities of different sectors including health and
social care, education, housing, leisure, employers and the third sector. In Chapter 2 we
explore the different dimensions of mental wellbeing from a theoretical perspective with a
view to using key ideas about flourishing, proportionate universalism and assets-based
approaches in developing practical approaches to commissioning for mental wellbeing.

The current context for commissioning is changing and arguably locating public health
within local authorities will enhance the opportunity to take action to address some of the
inequalities faced by different groups and thus promote population mental wellbeing (see
for example, Howarth, 2012, Appendix 1). Whilst this context is somewhat fluid at the
time of writing, the principles and process underpinning effective competent commissioning are well understood and thus Chapter 4 considers the commissioning process from the
perspective of improving population mental health. Using the rapidly developing evidence
base on the protective, risk and environmental factors associated with mental wellbeing
and the interventions that can promote mental wellbeing at an individual and social level
should assist in targeting effectively the interventions that are known to work. This will
demand the alignment of outcomes measures and information systems with strategies and
the goals of programmes and interventions, and in turn this requires a more explicit focus
on commissioning the mental wellbeing component of existing provision, better strategic
coordination of exiting activities and aspirations to improve mental wellbeing, and support for additional community activities and increased upstream investments.

Commissioning requires active engagement with the public and targeted groups, giving
them a voice to influence the availability of and access to interventions for physical and
mental wellbeing. Community engagement is also essential in tackling health inequalities
and to determine what assets are available in the community that can be used to ameliorate
the process of turning the deficits model around and we explore different models for community engagement in Chapter 5. Understanding and recognising diversity within communities and developing appropriate methods for engagement to determine interventions to
strengthen mental wellbeing will be essential. Too often in the past interventions that have
been shown to work in one place are slavishly copied somewhere else without sufficient
recognition of age, disability, ethnicity, religion or other important factors. Wellbeing for
black and minority ethnic communities may be constructed differently from that for the
majority community, and only by developing locally relevant interventions will we get cost-
effective, clinically relevant, psychologically appropriate and socially acceptable solutions.

Integration is a difficult concept, especially now (at the time of writing in January 2013)
as the government's attitude towards the market in health and social care may undermine
the best opportunities to integrate both vertically and horizontally around the citizen (the
patient, service user or client). Paradoxically health and wellbeing will only be fully secured
once systems and procedures are developed with the service user at the centre. This is one
of the contradictions of a public health approach in which the citizen is paramount: it
demands a universal focus on health and wellbeing whilst recognising the importance of
personalisation.

Health promotion is the process of enabling people to increase control over, and to
improve, their health. To reach a state of complete physical, mental and social wellbeing, an

individual or group must be able to identify and to realise aspirations, to satisfy needs and to change or cope with the environment. Health is, therefore, seen as a resource for every-day life, not the objective of living. Health is a positive concept emphasising social and personal resources, as well as physical capacities. Therefore, health promotion is not just the responsibility of the health sector, but goes beyond healthy lifestyles to wellbeing. In Chapters 6 to 9 we will consider in detail the interventions that lead to improved health and wellbeing in a number of areas and in Chapter 9 we consider promoting wellbeing for peo-ple with 'particular vulnerabilities', including people with a diagnosis of mental illness. And in the final chapter we will discover the population effects of all these interventions.

Whilst there is increasingly robust evidence for improved outcomes as a consequence of wellbeing interventions, much hangs on how these are implemented in real-life contexts. There is a tension between fidelity to the intervention as provided by the evidence base and the day to day contingencies that will influence outcomes at a local level. This is the focus for Chapter 10, where we explore how to implement best practice in local settings. In Chapter 11, we consider accountability for outcomes and approaches to evaluating and measuring outcomes including cost-effectiveness and the effectiveness of interventions measured against either professional or service user expectations. Our final chapter pro-vides a synthesis and concludes with a starting point in using this book as a resource to support improvements in population health and wellbeing.

1.8 Conclusion

Promoting health and wellbeing demands a composite strategy that draws on assets mod-els to generate solutions to individual health or illness problems, and recognises the value of a range of solutions for generating improved wellbeing from (in some cases) relatively complex multi-disciplinary interventions. Health, whether drawing on a deficit model or an assets model, is a foundation for flourishing but does not, of itself, generate wellbeing. A minimally adequate health is a necessary foundation for maximising wellbeing, but it is not sufficient. As we have discussed, wellbeing derives for a range of social, psycho-logical, emotional, spiritual, economic and familial contexts. Only by getting those right (or at least maximising them depending on circumstances) in the context of a health strategy that seeks equity of access and ability to benefit will it be possible to offer the best health and wellbeing available.

Notes

1 www.neweconomics.org/publications/measuring-well-being-in-policy; www.neweconomics.org/projects/five-ways-well-being (accessed 25 July 2012).
2 For further information see www.grossnationalhappiness.com for a discussion of Bhutan's GNH index.
3 And interdependence!
4 See for example Public Health England at www.lho.org.uk/LHO.Topics/Analytic_Tools/Health InequalitiesInterventionToolkit.aspx
5 i.e. is not fully constructed or determined by the intervention.
6 See also Zero to Three, at www.zerotothree.org (accessed 11 March 2013).

CHAPTER 2

Health and Wellbeing – Theoretical Considerations

There is no universally agreed definition of mental wellbeing and in this chapter we explore its different meanings and the key theoretical issues that underpin our approach. In particular, we consider theoretical approaches to the relationship between health and wellbeing and between mental wellbeing and mental illness. Wellbeing is an interplay of economic, social, cultural, community and environmental factors. Within this book we provide a considerable amount of detail on interventions that can be commissioned, and many of these require different organisations to work together at a national and local level to secure improvements in population wellbeing and tackle inequalities in health outcomes. Therefore, in this chapter we consider the relationship between income inequalities and wellbeing. Underpinning this focus on inequalities are values relating to equity and social justice and we therefore consider a values-based approach to commissioning that emphasises the importance of ethical reasoning alongside evidential reasoning. We conclude by considering the economic advantages to commissioning for health and wellbeing.

2.1 Introduction

We saw in Chapter 1 that our concern in this book is with health and wellbeing from the standpoint of positive mental health (not mental health read as mental illness) and positive wellbeing for all. Positive mental health includes what are often referred to as primary and secondary prevention. Whilst some of what we will cover in the book is about integrating 'services' (for example, bringing together services for people with depression, diabetes, cardiovascular disease and dementia) most of the book is about new ways to tackle chronic problems of poor wellbeing through the life course and to stimulate an interest in tackling a wide range of problems early, before the need for services arises. In doing this we need to think about what it is we want to achieve. Health is a contested subject; and wellbeing is seen by many as quite simply 'motherhood and apple pie' – what you get when everyone is more or less happy! We reject that idea as too simplistic, and substitute for it a robust focus on achieving good health based on well-researched and well-evidenced interventions.

2.2 Defining health and wellbeing

In 1978, at Alma Ata, the World Health Organization (WHO) passed a resolution that asked member governments to take urgent action on a number of critical matters. The first of these was a statement about health, which the conference strongly reaffirmed as:

> a state of complete physical, mental and social wellbeing, and not merely the absence of disease or infirmity, is a fundamental human right and that the attainment of the highest possible level of health is a most important world-wide social goal whose realization requires the action of many other social and economic sectors in addition to the health sector. (WHO, 1978)

That sentence, 'a state of complete physical, mental and social wellbeing, and not merely the absence of disease or infirmity', has been repeated many times, in many differing places, and formed the basis of 'Health for All by the Year 2000', the WHO programme for the 20 years to the end of the last century. As Burns (personal communication, 2012) has pointed out, however, the statement is, at face value, wrong. Health is not a 'state', to describe it in that way medicalises health; health is a dynamic process of interaction between the person and his or her body with the social, political, natural and economic environment. In other words health is situated and contingent on resources and the environmental context, in its broadest sense. So the WHO definition of health leaves many aspects to be agreed and defined.

No one has complete physical, mental and social wellbeing: as Tudor (1996: 42) observes, the WHO 'ambition of complete health perpetuates a grandiose and perfectionist view of the human condition'. Many people achieve wellbeing when living with a disability, or a continuing physical illness, or dementia. Where this definition was valuable though, leaving aside for the moment the important international dimension, was in setting in train work on health and wellbeing that is coming to fruition 35 years later. Whilst Alma Ata moved health beyond medicine, wellbeing is now seen as much more than health. Wellbeing incorporates health, happiness, income, welfare and much more. Michael Marmot's report on the social determinants of health and the debate that has encouraged shows just how far the world has come in the last 30 years.

If health promotion is the process of enabling populations to increase control over their health, then to reach a state of complete physical, mental and social wellbeing, an individual or group must be able to identify and to realise aspirations, to satisfy needs and to change or cope with the environment. Health is the foundation of a life worth living, a means to an end; it enables the achievement of goals and dreams. Health is a positive concept emphasising social and personal resources, as well as physical capacities. Health promotion – health as physical, mental and social wellbeing – is the responsibility of everyone, and demands a new way of thinking about positive mental health. Mental wellbeing is a similarly multi-dimensional concept and is the foundation for positive health and effective functioning for an individual and for a community. Five differing definitions can be found in the literature,[1] and we have placed them in a hierarchy with psychological wellbeing at the top (given its focus on mastery and control), and personal economic wellbeing at the bottom (Maslow's hierarchy of the building blocks of a decent life).

- Psychological wellbeing – a subjective term, and in that sense has a connection with subjective wellbeing – means a sense of *mastery and control, purpose and meaning*, including spirituality, creativity and positive functioning. It includes contentment, satisfaction with all elements of life, self-actualisation (a feeling of having achieved something with one's life), peace and happiness.[2]

- Emotional wellbeing is the ability to *understand the value of one's own emotions and use them positively*; a positive sense of wellbeing, a sense of self-esteem and self-respect that enables a person to function in society and meet the demands of everyday life; people in good emotional health have the ability to recover effectively from illness, change or misfortune.[3]
- Social and familial wellbeing refers to *positive relationships with others*, interdependence and social connectedness with others and society, and good family and personal relationships in which younger people grow to maturity with appropriate educational and parental support.
- Subjective wellbeing (SWB) refers to the way people experience and evaluate the quality of their lives and includes both emotional reactions and cognitive judgements, positive and negative affect, *happiness and life satisfaction*. Within subjective wellbeing we might include a sense of peace and contentment[4] (Jonas, 2005).
- Personal economic wellbeing means having sufficient resources for an acceptable life in which the usual goods of society are shared and accessible on the level of income available (in the literature, economic wellbeing is usually related to whole societies but is just as important to the individual and his or her family).

Of course, there will always be overlays and correspondences in any taxonomy, but in broad terms there is an association between the levels and the differing notions of wellbeing. On

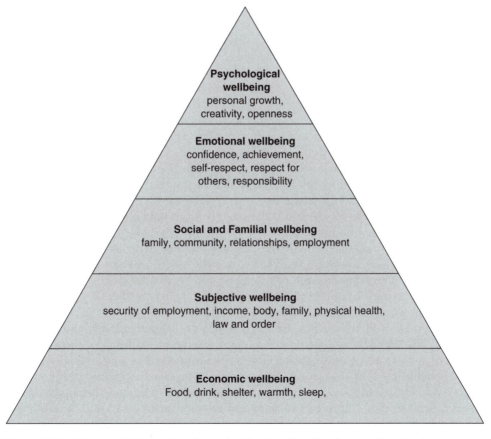

Figure 2.1 Maslow's hierarchy of need reflecting the five forms of wellbeing described above (redrawn from Maslow, 1943)

this model subjective wellbeing is more constrained than in some other models and describes the second level, one which is essential before a person can go on to feel love or belonging, emotional wellbeing and ultimately self-actualisation. But at the end of the day what really matters is the nature of wellbeing and how we can, through commissioned interventions, bring about improvements. Arising from this there are a number of questions to consider: what is the relationship between health and wellbeing? What is the relationship of mental wellbeing to mental illness: qualitatively the same or different? Are conceptions of wellbeing universally similar or do they differ across different cultures? What does all of this mean for evaluating and measuring improvements as a consequence of commissioning interventions?

a) The relationship between health and wellbeing

Our first question is to consider how health and wellbeing are partners. Is wellbeing something different from health? Or is health the underpinning of wellbeing? We know that being physically healthy is important for wellbeing, but it is not the only factor involved. Physical and emotional health are both important: having a good relationship with your spouse or partner, having friends or acquaintances on whom you can trust; being trusted in turn, and offering help to others; enjoying activities in your local community; and so on. Wellbeing is a multifaceted concept that concerns optimal functioning. From a review of research on mental wellbeing, Ryan and Deci (2001) identify two broad traditions – hedonic wellbeing and eudaimonic wellbeing. Hedonic wellbeing often refers to the subjective sense of wellbeing, notably happiness and life satisfaction, and is most usually termed subjective wellbeing. Eudaimonic wellbeing relates to the realisation of human potential and includes meaning, self-realisation and functioning in life and is often referred to as psychological wellbeing. Although these two concepts overlap, they are derived from two distinct traditions, both arising from Western philosophy – hedonism and eudaemonism. They differ fundamentally in terms of their views of what constitutes a good society and a good life (Ryan and Deci, 2001). Keyes (2006) has commented on the relative lack of focus on the social dimensions of an individual's functioning in life within the eudaimonic tradition of research. He has thus developed the concept of social wellbeing and proposed five dimensions – social coherence (whether a social life is seen as meaningful); social actualisation (whether society is seen as possessing potential for growth); social integration (a sense of belonging and acceptance by their communities); social acceptance (feel they accept other people); and social contribution (a sense of having something worthwhile to contribute) (Keyes 2006: 5).

In the literature, different terms are used, sometimes interchangeably and sometimes differently, but the distinction between a subjective sense of wellbeing (sometimes called happiness) and psychological wellbeing (a sense of purpose and meaning in life), is a useful one. This is illustrated by the paradox that someone who seeks happiness for him- or herself, will not find it, but the person who helps others will. In a study by Konow and Early, reported in 2008, they addressed two questions relevant to happiness and generosity: do more generous people report on average greater happiness, or subjective wellbeing, as measured by responses to various questionnaires? And, if the answer is in the affirmative, what is the causal relationship between generosity and happiness? They established that there was a positive correlation between generosity and happiness. What they found was that psychological wellbeing is the primary cause of both happiness and greater generosity.[5] Their results suggest that greater attention should be paid to policies that promote charitable donations, volunteerism, service education, and, more generally, community involvement, political action and social institutions that foster psychological wellbeing. None of these, you will note, are 'health' benefits, but nonetheless they promote 'health'.

b) The relationship between mental wellbeing and mental illness

Mental health in particular is used or viewed as a euphemism for mental illness. Nonetheless it raises an important theoretical question about the relationship between mental wellbeing (or positive mental health) and mental illness. There are two potential models for this relationship, as observed by Herron and Mortimer (1999). First, the bipolar or single continuum model reflects the view that mental wellbeing (positive mental health) exists at the opposing end of the same continuum as mental illness. The existence or degree of one is dependent on the existence, absence or degree of the other and mental wellbeing is therefore seen in terms of the absence or reduction of mental illness. Mental wellbeing has therefore been described as a secondary concept to mental illness; requiring prior knowledge of mental illness to be understood and inevitably viewed through 'the lens of mental illness' (Herron and Trent, 2000: 30).

The alternative model is the two or dual continua model, which suggests that mental health consists of two dimensions: mental health problems or mental illness and mental wellbeing (positive mental health) (Tudor, 1996; Keyes, 2007), as illustrated in Figure 2.2. Keyes introduced the concept of 'flourishing' to refer to people with good mental health

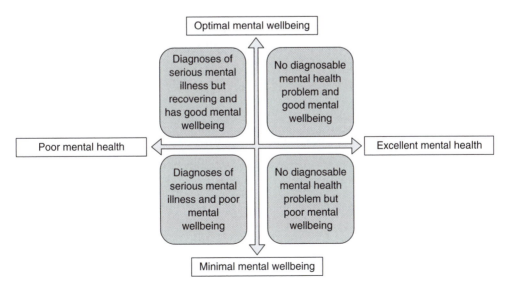

Figure 2.2 Dual continua model of positive mental health and wellbeing

Source: NHS Scotland, 2010, adapted from Tudor, 1996

and good mental wellbeing and has been adopted by different organisations to capture this sense that wellbeing is much more than the absence of mental health problems. Separating the definition of mental wellbeing from mental illness means that it is possible to focus on strengths rather than deficiencies, capacity rather than loss and growth rather than remediation (Herron and Trent, 2000), as consistent with the WHO definition.

There is emerging evidence to support the dual continua model – for example the data drawn from the Midlife in the United States (MIDUS) Survey, undertaken with English-speaking populations only. Furthermore, recent work from the positive psychology movement within clinical psychology has demonstrated the value of focusing on positive attributes of individual personality: (i) to tackle problems of psychopathology and (ii) as a health promoting and preventive strategy for enhancing positive thinking. Thus there is a move to an integrated approach to enhancing wellbeing (Joseph and Wood, 2010; Kashdan and Rottenberg, 2010; Wood et al., 2010; Wood and Tarrier, 2010). The general argument made by these writers is for an 'equally weighted focus on both positive and negative functioning' (Wood and Tarrier, 2010: 819) that integrates promotion and prevention. They suggest that 'positive characteristics', such as gratitude (Carver et al., 2010), optimism (Carver et al., 2010), and psychological flexibility (Kashdan and Rottenberg, 2010) assist in predicting and preventing disorders better than using 'pathological' characteristics.

The review by Wood and Tarrier (2010) is predicated on a theoretical position that explicates one of the paradoxes of health and wellbeing, i.e. that between 'health for all' as a 'positive' feature of wellbeing and prevention of mental disorder as a 'negative' feature (see below). In other words, the debate that we described at the beginning of the book – health is both physical, mental and social, but eudaimonic wellbeing is predicated largely on social and psychological health – and our predominant theme is psychological health and wellbeing, whether as a result of improved physical health, mental health or social functioning (Power, 2010).

Wood and Tarrier suggest that, 'positive and negative characteristics cannot logically be studied or changed in isolation as (a) they interact to predict clinical outcomes, (b) characteristics are neither "positive" or "negative", with outcomes depending on specific situation and concomitant goals and motivations, and (c) positive and negative wellbeing often exist on the same continuum' (p.819). In principle this does not sound persuasive. Whilst we can understand that positive and negative features interact in sometimes complex ways, Keyes' (2007) article supports the two continua model of mental health and illness, and the benefits of flourishing to individuals and society. We will see this again in Chapter 10 when we consider the eudaimonic and hedonic aspects of flourishing. Mental health is much more than the absence of mental illness; it is what makes life enjoyable, productive and fulfilling, and it contributes to social capital and economic development in societies (Keyes, 1998). Mentally healthy adults[6] reported 'the fewest missed days of work … the healthiest psychosocial functioning (i.e. low helplessness, clear goals in life, high resilience, and high intimacy), the lowest risk of cardiovascular disease, the lowest number of chronic physical diseases with age, the fewest health limitations of activities of daily living, and lower health care utilization' (Keyes, 2007: 95).

Many of these features are aspects of physical health. Unhappily, the likelihood that a person would be flourishing is low, at around one fifth of the adult population. This is unsurprising. In practice, mental health as 'fully flourishing' demands a great deal of the individual and society and thus of the interventions to improve that individual's life chances. Flourishing includes some or all of the following: emotional wellbeing with positive affect, satisfaction with life overall, positive self-attitudes and awareness, commitment to personal growth with a life that has direction and meaning, being able to form warm and trusting relationships with positive social functioning in their own daily activities, with a sense of belonging and being useful to and valued by society and others (Keyes, 2007: extracted from Table 1, p. 98). How many can aspire to that ideal, which is contingent upon social, environmental and political constraints? In practice we will set the bar quite a bit lower when we come to evaluate the outcomes from health and wellbeing interventions.

c) Cultural differences in the conception of mental wellbeing

The research suggests that there may be differences between different cultures in terms of not only the language that is used, but also how wellbeing is conceptualised and therefore the basis for evaluations of wellbeing. This is not to reify culture but to indicate that there are different frames of reference used by people from different cultural backgrounds and that this will be an important consideration in developing health and wellbeing strategies in an increasingly diverse and multicultural Britain.

The distinction in the literature is typically drawn between individualist cultures (i.e. Anglo-American or Western) and collectivist cultures (i.e. Eastern) and these are used as ideal types to characterise different frames of reference. In reality many people will draw on more than one frame of reference, reflecting their heritage and educational experience. Nonetheless, this distinction cautions against assuming conceptual equivalence, i.e. that the concept of mental wellbeing has the same meaning across different cultures. Kleinman (1987) identified this risk as a categorical fallacy where disease classifications are developed for one cultural group then applied to another. There has been relatively little empirical work to explore whether mental wellbeing constructs are equally applicable across different populations (Cheng and Chan, 2005). However, conceptions of subjective and psychological wellbeing have been criticised for deriving from philosophical traditions (hedonia and eudaimonia) that reflect Western, and possibly middle- and upper-class definitions of what it means to live a full and satisfying life (Keyes et al., 2002). On the other hand, Eastern perspectives may emphasise connection to others, meeting obligations and achieving fulfilment through carefully managed social ties, which reflect an integrated view of the physical, spiritual and emotional aspects of health and illness in sharp contrast with mind–body dualism of Western philosophies (Belippa, 1991).

These conceptual differences are illustrated by research both in the UK and other contexts. For example, happiness has been identified as widely used within Chinese communities but has a fuller meaning than positive mood and the absence of negative mood as typically found in literature following the US school of thought (Ryan and Deci, 2001). Lu and Shih (1997) describe the Chinese conception of happiness as including material abundance, physical health, virtuous and peaceful life and relief from death anxiety. Older Chinese people in Manchester used the term happiness and defined it in terms of being content with life, absence of worry, family welfare, social connections and freedom from physical illness (Chan et al., 2007). Liu et al. (2005) observed that traditional Chinese values stress collectivism, cooperation, modesty, courtesy, academic achievement, in-group harmony and hierarchical relationships. They contrast this with Western culture, with its emphasis on individualism, competition, independence and equality of relationships. However, it is also erroneous to assume that non-Western views are homogenous. For example, Newbigging et al. (2008) explored conceptions of wellbeing by Chinese and Pakistani communities. Whilst Chinese communities used the term happiness, members of Pakistani communities were initially more likely to describe mental wellbeing in terms of the absence of mental illness but also referred to a 'peaceful mind'. They found that both communities emphasised family wellbeing, spiritual wellbeing and material wellbeing alongside the importance of social roles and connectedness. These findings, and the suggestion that there are age and gender differences in conceptions of wellbeing reinforce the importance of engagement and co-production.

Wellbeing therefore has an ontological nature and this raises questions about the appropriateness of measures of mental wellbeing outcomes. In other words, the wellbeing of a person should be based on an evaluation of the kind of life he or she is living, or wants to lead. Defining, describing, measuring and understanding that life relates to whatever we call wellbeing. As discussed above, this raises questions that have personal, cultural, social, ethical and political dimensions. Differing theoretical positions will also provide differing answers. As van Ootegem and Spillemaeckers (2010: 384) suggest, '[F]or some, personal wellbeing is (only) about poverty, basic needs or resources. Others hold that wellbeing has to do (only) with happiness or with spirituality or mental fitness'. Still others have ideas of wellbeing that include such matters as family life, personal success, aspirations achieved, health maintained and diseases beaten.

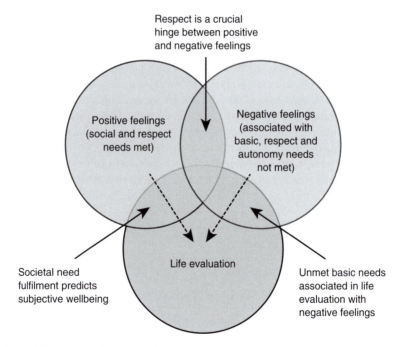

Figure 2.3 Life evaluation based on positive and negative feelings (based on Tay and Diener, 2011)

Tay and Diener (2011) took samples of people from 123 countries in order to understand the association between the fulfilment of needs and subjective wellbeing. Need fulfilment was consistently associated across all cultures with subjective wellbeing. Life evaluation was most associated with having basic needs met; positive feelings were most associated with social and respect needs; and negative feelings with basic, respect, and autonomy needs going unmet.

Figure 2.3 suggests that living in a flourishing society is desirable for wellbeing (Tay and Diener, 2011); or perhaps, as the present political and economic situation shows, it is possible to forget the macro-economic context of society if other aspects are promoted and sustained (such as, at the time of writing, the Olympic Games).

Nonetheless, Figure 2.3 also suggests that subjective wellbeing is fickle and can change (or be changed) quite rapidly if people's perception of prosperity is denied. Indeed, whilst achievements of social needs were more or less consistent between countries, realisation of basic needs was dependent on individual country conditions. Community resilience is an important feature of overall wellbeing. For example, some 75% of British people told an ONS survey in early 2012 that they were happy and satisfied with life.[7]

2.3 Social Determinants of Health

a) Inequality and inequity

In their book, *The Spirit Level*, Wilkinson and Pickett (2009) demonstrate that there is more or less direct correlation between health and social problems and income inequality in differing countries, but a weak correlation or no correlation at all between the index and average income. The index of health and social problems is based on the factors in Figure 2.4 below.

When the index calculated for each of a number of 'Western' countries (including Australia and Japan) and plotted against average income, it produces a graph onto which can be superimposed a relatively straight regression line. The most significant outlier is the USA which has both high income inequality and a higher than expected index of health and social problems. Wilkinson and Pickett show that child wellbeing, for example, is better in more equal societies, as are levels of trust, whilst mental illness is lower. Dr Lynn

Life expectancy	Teenage births
Ability at maths and literacy	Trust
Infant mortality	Obesity
Homicides	Mental illness and drug and alcohol dependency
Imprisonment	Social mobility

Figure 2.4   Inequalities in health and social problems. Factors used to create an index
Source: Wilkinson and Pickett, *The Spirit Level* (2009)

Friedli in a report for the World Health Organization (2008) highlights the emotional and cognitive effects of high levels of social status differentiation. As Friedli writes: 'greater inequality heightens status competition and status insecurity across all income groups and among adults and children' (Friedli, 2009: iii). It is therefore the distribution of economic and social resources which is important in explaining health and other outcomes and this analysis underscores the work of the Marmot Review (2010), which we turn to in the next section.

b) *Fair Society, Healthy Lives*

Mental wellbeing is influenced by a complex interplay of factors at an individual, social and community level (see, for example, DH, 2009a). The focus has increasingly shifted to the role played by inequalities and Sir Michael Marmot's report on the social determinants of health has been enormously influential. The report, *Fair Society, Healthy Lives: A Strategic Review of Health Inequalities in England Post-2010* (Marmot, 2010) has become a touchstone for further work. The final report concluded that reducing health inequalities would require action on six policy objectives:

1 Give every child the best start in life.
2 Enable all children, young people and adults to maximise their capabilities and have control over their lives.
3 Create fair employment and good work for all.
4 Ensure a healthy standard of living for all.
5 Create and develop healthy and sustainable places and communities.
6 Strengthen the role and impact of ill-health prevention.

We can see that these six policy objectives contain many more than six action items; each is a composite of individual, potentially large, work programmes, and will be challenging especially at times of austerity and funding reductions. However, we will argue (see Chapters 3 and 11) that the cost reductions in the UK and other European countries is an opportunity to try new ways of tackling health and health care, of which the programme outlined in the Marmot Review is ambitious and achievable. Not only are there opportunities to implement the findings of the review, but the review has catalysed other organisations to develop similar discrete, related programmes of activity. For example, the Global Health Equity Foundation (www.ghef.org) is mapping health inequities and developing a comparative methodology for determining strategies to reduce equity gaps in various countries; it will in 2013–14 establish an international action programme in six or seven countries where there are serious health problems.

The World Health Organization established a Commission on Social Determinants of Health between 2005 and 2008 to 'support countries and global health partners address the social factors leading to ill health and inequities'. From an international perspective, the overarching recommendations of the Commission were to:

• improve daily living conditions;
• tackle the inequitable distribution of power, money and resources;
• measure and understand the problem and assess the impact of action.[8]

We shall consider the WHO Commission on Social Determinants of Health, the Marmot Review and a number of other initiatives later (in Chapter 3). In addition, the World Health Organization European Region has announced that they are commissioning Professor Marmot to conduct a two-year European Review (which will be almost complete when this book is published). The purpose of this Review will be to review health inequalities and their social determinants across Europe, with a view to developing policies, building capacity and recommending practical steps to address the social determinants of health.

At this point, however, it is worth noting that Marmot's approach is not without its critics. As we have seen, Marmot argued that societies should focus on reducing health inequalities, through achieving vital changes to make society fairer (Marmot, 2010). Marmot advances two reasons: first, that the primary goal of government policy should be to reduce or remove the socio-economic gradient in health; and second, that health outcomes are largely determined by social factors and to reduce health inequalities we must first reduce social inequality (Canning and Bowser, 2010: 1223). But Canning and Bowser take a different view. They argue that a better goal would be to improve overall health, income levels and socio-economic outcomes for the most disadvantaged in society, and that the way to do this is using direct health interventions, 'particularly interventions that improve health in early childhood that can have long-term benefits in physical and cognitive development'. Their rationale is that health improvements lead to improvements in socio-economic outcomes, rather than that improved socio-economic conditions lead to improved health. This, as Canning and Bowser suggest (p.1223), 'revers[es] the direction of causality put forward in the Marmot reports'. Although they take a diametrically opposite view on causality, their implementation programme is remarkably similar to Marmot's. Direct health interventions, particularly with children, are in their view mechanisms for improving *both* health and socio-economic outcomes.

In 2010, we put forward a not dissimilar observation on the practical interventions. In discussing the needs of children and adolescents we proposed that the health promotion slogan should be 'focus on children, start with adults' (Heginbotham and Newbigging, 2010). By investing resources into achieving good prenatal, perinatal and postnatal care, ensuring that young mothers and fathers have the necessary skills and resources to deal with childcare effectively through universal parenting programmes, and intervening early with postnatal depression and psychosis, we believed it would be possible to reduce the worst implications of childhood trauma. For example, Friedli and Parsonage (2007) estimated that the savings to be achieved from spending £210 million on UK parent training programmes for parents of children with conduct disorder (5% of the childhood population), could be as much as £5.2 billion over the following 20 years, by obviating treatments for the worst effects of the disorders prevented, reductions in a range of undesirable behaviours and improved adolescent and adult health.

c) Proportionate universalism

A key concept that Marmot has introduced into the debate is that of proportionate universalism.

> To reduce the steepness of the social gradient in health, actions must be universal, but with a scale and intensity that is proportionate to the level of disadvantage. We call this proportionate universalism. (Marmot, 2010: 15)

Whilst there is good evidence for universal interventions – i.e. those that are not targeted on specific at-risk groups but are applied to the whole population – they have been criticised for benefiting those sections of the population most able to benefit thus perpetuating inequalities they are designed to attenuate. They also do not take adequate account of diversity in the population; different segments of the population may respond in different ways to similar interventions or require interventions to be adapted or take account of specific identity-related issues. On the other hand, targeting interventions can be criticised on two broad grounds: that some, perhaps many, people miss out on the intervention when they might have benefited, and that prior judgements have been made about who is most at risk. Only a balanced or proportionate universalism – that is, a sensible balance across increasingly targeted groups of increasingly disadvantaged populations – can achieve the best of both worlds and this is discussed in more detail in Chapters 4 and 5.

2.4 Values-based commissioning

In a helpful paper, Carter et al. (2011: 465) proposed a 'new' approach to guide health promotion practice. Health promotion, they suggest, should 'draw on two related systems of reasoning: an evidential system and an ethical system'. More interestingly they offer the proposal that the 'concepts, values, and procedures' should be made explicit. We agree: values are the other side of the coin of evidence. Evidence-based medicine is one half of the field; the other half is values. Values-based practice is not another theoretical category with little relevance to health promotion and prevention. It is fundamental to those subjects. Values-basing is about the processes that can be applied to the social determinants of health, and all forms of health promotion and prevention, anywhere.

Values-based health and wellbeing describes the theoretical and practical demands on citizens and health care workers of using stated values to achieve an improved process for filtering the available evidence to achieve improved outcomes for citizens, patients and service users.[9] Health and social care are values-driven as well as evidence-driven enterprises. Although there has increasingly been an expectation that the evidence base of health and wellbeing strategies should be made fully explicit, the corresponding values base has by and large been left largely implicit. Values-based health and wellbeing thus complements evidence-based methodologies by providing a skills base and other support processes for working with differences of values that are held by all those engaged in making decisions to commission one or other health and wellbeing strategy.

The challenge of values-basing everything we do is four-fold. First, there are many values, some of which are not usually engaged in health promoting, wellbeing and preventive strategies, though they may be part of the wider culture from which citizens, patients and service users are drawn. Understanding those values is necessary to ensure that everyone and especially minority groups and cultures are given due weight in all discussions about health and wellbeing strategies. Second, values can be written in various ways, but are usually normative statements that affirm how things should be or ought to be, which things are good or bad, or which actions are right or wrong. Values are the principles with which we lead our lives; some are held more firmly than others, but everyone has them!

Third, values cover many aspects of life which impinge directly on health and wellbeing strategies; these may not be our most pressing concerns but sometimes they become much more important for short periods or for small but significant matters. Fourth, values

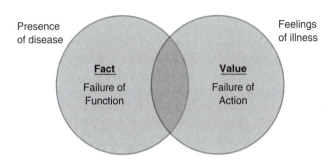

Presence
of disease

Fact

Failure of
Function

Feelings
of illness

Value

Failure of
Action

Figure 2.5   The fact–value relationship

concern the felt aspects of wellness or illness, as opposed to the factual issues of disease; values are an essential component of any serious discussion about health and wellbeing, about prevention and health promotion, about mental health as well as physical health. Fulford (2004) has demonstrated the importance of values as reflecting the felt aspects of illness in comparison to the facts of disease (see Figure 2.5).

However, Carter et al. (2011: 468) suggest that 'health promotion thinking must be responsive to particular situations – it cannot be universal'. Our approach on the other hand is to emphasise the important universal aspect of *all* health and wellbeing strategies, whilst recognising the situated nature of interventions and the influence of contextual factors on action. We do not argue that everything that is 'produced' in each relevant strategy area should be universal but we take the idea of proportionate universalism from the Marmot Review report. Proportionate universalism offers a way to provide a health and wellbeing intervention to all, regardless of their status, and to make subsequent interventions more targeted depending on the requirements of the group. Similarly, the NHS is a universal service, funded out of taxation. It may not be as comprehensive as we might wish but it is available to anyone, regardless of ability to pay at the time of need. No one need be reluctant to use the service because they do not have the means.

2.5 Drivers of wellbeing

We need to understand the main drivers of wellbeing. If, for example, wellbeing was not related to health states, then we would be acting unethically to use health funding to develop interventions to promote wellbeing. Alternately, if wellbeing is a feature of good mental and/or physical health we will then feel much better in using health money to achieve improvements in health as a proxy for improving wellbeing. Wellbeing is a complex amalgam of many factors, of which health is a significant component. According to Fischer and Boer (2011), where a person has good health (i.e. if we control for 'health' by assuming good health) then, globally, individualism has been canvassed as more important than money in sustaining wellbeing. But this begs the question of how we measure wellbeing. Individual wellbeing is the 'subjective assessment of one's life including emotional reactions to personal events, mood states and any judgment concerning satisfaction and fulfilment in various domains of life' (Fischer and Boer, 2011: 164). Fischer and Boer examined data on wellbeing from 63 independent country datasets on over 420,000 individuals; wellbeing was measured using information on the lack of psychological health, anxiety and stress measures. Their claim is that, 'despite some emerging non-linear trends … *the overall pattern strongly suggests that greater individualism is consistently associated with more wellbeing*' (2011: Abstract, emphasis added). They suggest that income and wealth will only influence wellbeing though the way they impact on individualism.

Unfortunately, whilst this may contain some kernel of truth, individualism and wealth (or income) are not independent variables. In whatever way we define wellbeing, a number of authors have shown there is a decrease in wellbeing, with more depression and stress, as individual freedom, autonomy and choice increase (Fischer and Boer, 2011). Fischer and Boer's reading of the literature suggests that the relation between wealth, or individualism, and wellbeing breaks down into three fairly distinct zones: first, when people have little or no choice this is associated with negative wellbeing; second, increased choice encourages feelings of economic freedom and the opportunity to satisfy basic needs; third, as people become better off, they become unable to use all the information available and suffer from difficulties in making choices, which are associated with negative wellbeing. In the graph of wealth versus wellbeing in Figure 2.6, we see Fischer and Boer assume that it is possible to draw a curvilinear regression line through the points on the graph of wealth and (negative) wellbeing (black line).

We think it is possible to take a different perspective. We can detect three separate graphs in the one chart. On the left there is a striking reduction in wellbeing as wealth increases from low levels; in the middle there are roughly static levels of negative wellbeing as wealth increases; and on the right a clear indication that, beyond a certain level of wealth, wellbeing is not dependent on wealth (or individualism) at all but on some other factor. In the second graph on individualism and wellbeing, the countries in the middle group show a greater scatter and (ironically) a correspondingly stronger regression line supporting the contention that individualism and wellbeing are positively correlated. However, close examination suggests that another undetected variable is responsible. This may be culture, social structure, political factors, family structure or originating factors. As these countries were newly emergent from Soviet hegemony when the data was obtained, it is likely that, as they become more Westernised, the results will change.

One aspect of this that demands explanation is that Fischer and Boer's graphs are not linear, at least not in the central section, which does not accord with the explanation offered by Wilkinson and Pickett in *The Spirit Level* (2009). Their contention is that inequality of income drives inequality in almost every other factor or a fairly linear correlation. The difference is probably in the construction of the variables and the number of differing domains of data. Where there is no or little choice then the notion of a linear correlation holds. Similarly at the higher end where there appears to be an almost vertical straight line relationship between countries. In the middle there is an area of latent wellbeing that does not appear to accord with the correlation put forward by Wilkinson and Pickett (2009).

As a final note on this fascinating debate, we turn to Fischer and Boer's remarks on the interplay of wealth and individualism: 'It appears plausible', they say, 'that increased wealth leads to more autonomy and freedom. Increasing wealth in a society may influence wellbeing, primarily through allowing citizens to experience greater autonomy and freedom in their daily lives' (2011: 177). In other words, increased wealth increases choice and individualistic expression. If this is so, what can we take from Fischer and Boer's interesting analysis? The main conclusion must be that the factors used to describe and quantify 'wellbeing' are too restrictive, and the factors involved in quantifying 'individualism' are too complex and have not been made explicit.

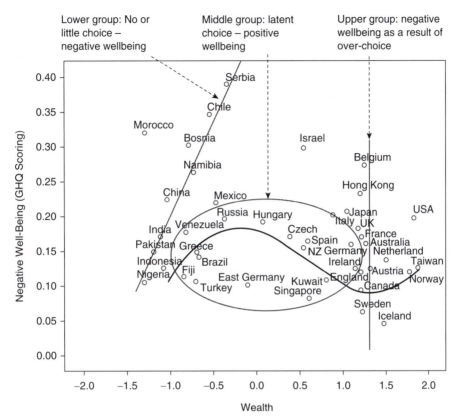

Three regions: left hand line represents those countries where income is too low for it to improve wellbeing, and indeed wellbeing suffers as income rises a little; the oval area (especially those countries of the old Soviet bloc) indicates those countries in which wellbeing is improved as a result of latent or potential choice; and the right hand line suggest those countries (c. f. The spirit level) in which wellbeing is not related to higher wealth or higher levels of choice. In this latter area there must be another factor at play, which the authors of the original paper have not captured. Original diagram amended from Fischer and Boer, 2011: Relationships between wealth and General Health Questionnaire (GHQ) scores (model 6a); higher scores on GHQ indicated greater psychological distress, anxiety, and social dysfunction. East Germany = German Democratic Republic; NZ = New Zealand; UK = United Kingdom; USA = United States of America.

Figure 2.6 An analysis of Fischer and Boer's wealth–wellbeing graph

As with so much epidemiological evidence it is the confounders, biases and interdependence of variables that get in the way. Having said that, extending individualism as empowerment may improve wellbeing under certain conditions, at particular points in history; how that message might be implemented, and whether it is a culturally bound analysis will be considered later. One problem with these results is adaptation effects, in which citizens discount the value of available wellbeing so that any additional wellbeing does not add to the previous total. Wellbeing also appears to fluctuate periodically: positive changes in one of the life domains (except health) in a previous period are associated with decreasing wellbeing in the present period (Binder and Coad, 2010). Binder and Coad go on to say that 'increases in … income are also associated with subsequent decreases in wellbeing, pointing to an explanation in terms of hedonic adaptation or rising aspiration levels' (p.353).

2.6 Relationship between lifestyle and health care costs: the economics of interventions

Demographic changes over the decade 2010–2020 have begun to place very significant pressures on local authorities and health agencies. This will be especially true of the growing numbers of older people, one fifth of whom over the age of 80 will have dementia and another fifth will be unable to carry out the usual activities of daily living. Without investment in preventive strategies, statutory authorities' budgets will be unable to cope. There is thus another imperative – the demographic time-bomb – that makes investment in this area essential. Commissioning public health and wellbeing offers potential savings by strengthening protective factors and reducing risk factors, with implications for health and social care usage elsewhere. Lower health care utilisation is another likely result so that investment in wellbeing interventions will have positive impacts in other parts of the health system.

There is evidence that mental wellbeing can reduce risks to health through influencing positive health behaviours, such as reductions in alcohol and substance use (see Chapter 6 for a fuller discussion); increase life expectancy, provide protection from coronary heart disease (CHD) and improve health outcomes from a range of long-term conditions (e.g. diabetes or Alzheimer's disease) (see Chapter 8 for a fuller discussion); reduce health inequalities – both physical and mental health – and impact positively on the social determinants of health; and, reduce mental health problems, especially depression and anxiety, and the consequences of mental illness or distress. There is also evidence that good mental health is associated with improved educational attainment and subsequent occupation and wellbeing outcomes; safer communities with less crime; improved worksite productivity and employee retention; and reduced sickness absence from work.

All these benefits have economic advantages. There are three main economic reasons for ensuring a greater focus on whole population health promotion and prevention strategies alongside early diagnosis and intervention. These are:

1   Improved physical health leads to reductions in both short-term and longer-term costs to health purchasers and providers, and improved mental health leads to savings in areas other than health.
2   Primary preventive strategies ensure that people remain healthy longer and identify disease early when costs are lower and prognoses are better (for both mental or physical health problems).
3   Improved mental health leads to savings in both mental health and physical health care costs. Resilience and recovery programmes (secondary and tertiary prevention) ensure that the effects of mental illness is minimised, and there are direct savings due to reduced use of mental health services as improved population mental health reduces risk of mental illness. Better mental health also reduces risk behaviour such as alcohol and smoking.

Determining the economics of health and wellbeing interventions requires a complex programme that includes the following. We need to know:

- first, what we mean by wellbeing as it relates to health (as we have discussed in the first part of this chapter) – in other words a rigorous operational **definition** (or definitions for differing areas of health) of wellbeing to allow a robust analysis of the data on wellbeing interventions;
- second, the necessary **process** requirements for establishing an intervention – in other words, all aspects of the intervention including the costs of actives to support implementation;

- third, what improvement in wellbeing is achievable with the various interventions possible, the **measurement** techniques available and what **evidence** we have of efficacy; and
- fourth, the **costs** estimated as accurately as possible.

Addressing the social determinants of health will inevitably mean addressing the discriminatory and socio-economic reasons that lead to a reduction in wellbeing for some groups. Programmes must be culturally relevant and appropriate and should address the needs of communities in ways that can be assimilated locally and be relevant to the needs of all parts of the community – respecting diversity in language, religion, ethnicity, disability, age, sexuality and income. Wellbeing concerns enhancements to social justice and reduction of social inequalities. Wellbeing is multi-factorial and is amenable to action for improvement at three interconnected levels:

- Structural – initiatives to reduce discrimination and inequalities and promote access to education, meaningful employment, affordable housing, health, social and other services for the whole population and simultaneously support those who are vulnerable.
- Community – increases in social support, social inclusion and participation in local communities and improving neighbourhood environments with anti-bullying strategies in schools, workplace health programmes, community safety schemes and childcare and self-help networks.
- Individual – increasing emotional resilience through interventions designed to promote self-esteem, life and coping skills such as parenting skills and communication skills, and personal control.

One of those who has done a lot of work on this is Martin Knapp at the London School of Economics and University of Kent, who with colleagues was asked by the Department of Health in 2010 to consider a number of (mental) health related interventions. We put 'mental' in parentheses as some of the interventions were physical interventions that had mental health consequences.

Box 2.1   Examples of wellbeing initiatives investigated by Knapp et al. (2011)

1 Health visiting and reducing postnatal depression

2 Parenting interventions for the prevention of persistent conduct disorders

3 School-based social and emotional learning (SEL) programmes to prevent conduct problems in childhood

4 School-based interventions to reduce bullying

5 Early detection for psychosis

6 Early intervention for psychosis

7 Screening and brief intervention in primary care for alcohol misuse

8 Workplace screening for depression and anxiety disorders

(Continued)

> *(Continued)*
>
> 9　Promoting wellbeing in the workplace
>
> 10　Debt and mental health
>
> 11　Population level suicide awareness training and intervention
>
> 12　Bridge safety measures for suicide prevention
>
> 13　Collaborative care for depression in individuals with Type 2 diabetes
>
> 14　Tackling medically unexplained symptoms
>
> 15　Befriending of older adults

Knapp and collaborators considered 15 interventions for which there was reasonable evidence of effectiveness and cost (Box 2.1). These cover only a small subset of the wider health and wellbeing programmes in which we are interested. For example, as we will see in Chapter 6, points 1–4 above are the precursor for a range of adolescent and adult health problems; similarly in Chapter 8 we will investigate the inter-relationship between diabetes (point 13 above) with depression, obesity (and exercise) and dementia. In Chapter 11 we will look in a little more detail at the cost-effectiveness estimates and consider why some interventions do not score well on cost-effectiveness measures. A further grouping brings together Parkinson's disease (PD), multiple sclerosis, rheumatoid arthritis, diabetes and Alzheimer's disease (dementia) for which there is evidence of inter-relatedness from genome wide association studies (GWAS) and interactome[10] investigations. In each of these subjects we will be concerned mainly with what we know about or can discern from the literature about relevant and focused health promotion and prevention activity and where we may get economically relevant information in order to support economically justified implementation.

To take just three areas of mental health care, McCrone et al. (2008) estimate that the costs are projected to increase as follows: those of dementia from £14.9 billion to £34.8 billion between 2007 (the baseline of the study) and 2026; the costs of anxiety related disorders from £8.9 billion to £14.2 billion; and the costs of depression from £7.5 billion to £12.2 billion. Similarly, the direct treatment costs of diabetes (without factoring in the costs of related disorders such as depression and dementia) are forecast to increase from £9.8 billion in 2012 to £16.9 billion over the next 25 years to 2035.[11] From a preventive and health promotion angle, weight and obesity are the most significant aspects that need effective interventions. We will look at this in some detail in the chapter on diabetes, including ways of reducing the incidence and prevalence of the disease (Hex et al., 2012).[12]

2.7 Conclusion

This chapter has covered a lot of theoretical and policy ground. What we mean by wellbeing has been explored and we have noted that it is more than solely subjective wellbeing, although this depends on how we define wellbeing. Perhaps more importantly we have shown that wellbeing is constructed on a number of differing premises and is influenced, and indeed undermined, by discrimination, inequality, deprivation, lack of social justice and lack of self-esteem. Conversely positive mental health and wellbeing can be achieved by tackling these problem areas through affirmative action and interventions that promote health, social status and wellbeing, prevent illness (physical and mental) and achieve wellbeing for people with diagnosed mental health problems.

Notes

1 In practice there are many differing definitions in the literature that overlap and duplicate each other. The five given here are compounds of various definitions in the literature.

2 http://answers.google.com/answers/threadview/id/32811.html (accessed 4 August 2012).

3 www.belongto.org/resource.aspx?contentid=4574 (accessed 4 August 2012).

4 Happiness (and subjective wellbeing) is a combination of life satisfaction and reflects the times when a person feels 'up' or 'down' (Diener, 1984). Diener at al. (1999) claim that subjective wellbeing 'tends to be stable over time' and is strongly related to personality. There is evidence that health and SWB may influence each other, as positive health is often associated with greater contentment, and various studies have found that constructive emotions have a beneficial influence on health (Diener and Chan, 1984; Okun et al., 1984; Diener, 2000; Steel et al., 2008). But whether SWB is as all-encompassing as is claimed, given the other ways in which wellbeing is defined, is open to question.

5 As the researchers conclude, the experimental method of this inquiry permits anonymity measures designed to minimise subject misrepresentation of intrinsic generosity (e.g., due to social approval motives) and of actual happiness (e.g., because of social desirability biases) and produces a rich data set with multiple measures of subjective, psychological and material wellbeing. The results of this and other studies raise the question of whether greater attention should be paid to the potential benefits (beyond solely the material ones) of policies that promote charitable donations, volunteerism, service education and, more generally, community involvement, political action and social institutions that foster psychological wellbeing (Konow and Early, 2008).

6 Keyes (1998) describes 'completely' mental healthy adults. We have deleted 'completely' as we do not believe anyone is ever 'completely' mentally (or physically) healthy. However the broad position Keyes takes is helpful in demonstrating once again the dichotomy between, and yet the continuum of, preventive strategies for mental illness/disorder, and the positive strategies for flourishing that have twin objectives: encouraging flourishing in people with mental disorder (what we generally refer to here as 'recovery') and flourishing for those without any diagnosable mental illness.

7 About three-quarters of people were satisfied with life, according to a study to measure wellbeing by the Office for National Statistics (ONS). The survey of 4,200 people asked respondents to rank from 0 to 10 how satisfied they were and how anxious they felt the previous day. When asked about how satisfied they were, 76% rated themselves as 7 out of 10, where 10 was completely satisfied and 0 was not satisfied at all. When asked how happy they felt the previous day, the results showed 73% rated themselves as 7 or more out of 10. To the question about leading a worthwhile life, 78% of respondents rated themselves 7 or more out of 10. The ONS added four questions to the UK household survey, which took place between April and August 2012, The questions included:
Overall, how satisfied are you with your life nowadays?
Overall, how happy did you feel yesterday?
Overall, how anxious did you feel yesterday?

Overall, to what extent do you feel the things you do in your life are worthwhile? Source: www.bbc.co.uk/news/uk-15989841 (accessed 5 August 2012).

 8 These points are addressed at www.who.int/social_determinants/thecommission/en/ (accessed 11 March 2011).

 9 We will use the term citizens to refer to all those to whom the health and wellbeing programmes are directed, and it will be taken to include patients, service users and citizens unless otherwise stated.

10 In molecular biology an 'interactome' is defined as the whole set of molecular interactions in cells. Specifically it means physical interactions amongst molecules but can also mean indirect interactions amongst genes, i.e. genetic interactions. It is usually displayed as a directed graph.

11 The study also reported that the costs of treating diabetes complications (including kidney failure, nerve damage, stroke, blindness and amputation) are expected to almost double from £7.7 billion currently to £13.5 billion by 2035/36.

12 See, for example, a *Daily Mail* article citing the report, www.dailymail.co.uk/health/article-2134821/Diabetes-bankrupt-NHS-spending-avoidable-say-experts.html (accessed 26 April 2012).

CHAPTER 3

Equity in Health and Wellbeing – Gaps and Gradients

Developments of health and wellbeing are dependent on two critical features: transformational thinking that places an emphasis on holistic person-centred health and social care; and achievement of equity in health and social care outcomes. In this chapter we will review the second of these two features and describe, from an international perspective, how equity gaps and gradients can be tackled. Proposals derived from the World Health Organization's Commission on the Social Determinants of Health (CSDH) are juxtaposed with other mechanisms for dealing with equity concerns, including the Urban HEART instrument advanced by the WHO Asia Pacific region (WHO, 2005). Global challenges are described including, but not exclusively, the effects and consequences of climate change for wellbeing, in addition to mechanisms to reduce the implications of inequality.

3.1 Introduction

As we saw in Chapter 2, a great deal of theoretical and practical work has been done by Sir Michael Marmot and colleagues internationally in the WHO Commission on Social Determinants of Health and by Marmot and UK colleagues in the report *Fair Society, Healthy Lives* (Marmot, 2010). In this chapter we will apply some of the learning from those reports and from other publications in considering the implications of equity gaps and equity gradients in the areas of (mental) health and wellbeing in the UK. Equity Gap Analysis (EGA) offers the opportunity to understand the principal factors contributing to problems of health inequalities and strategies for improving equity within individual countries (and between countries). The assignment is made more difficult as health equity is multi-factorial; generating sensible and appropriate comparisons between differing conditions or geographical areas depends on finding variables that are commensurable. This may mean that only a high-level analysis is possible in many cases, or that countries will have to be considered in clusters with similar sets of factors. Nonetheless there are techniques and approaches that may be of value to those commissioning interventions which may assist in ensuring the greatest efficiency and effectiveness of the investment.

Fortunately, the task is made easier by the focus that has come onto health equity, and in particular the social determinants of health, during the last six or seven years, and especially in the number of relevant research papers published since 2010. In addition to the Marmot Review[1] in the UK with the catalyst that has given to public health at a time of transition to local authority responsibility, there have been a number of useful papers produced by the World Health Organization globally and regionally, and by individual countries and groups of countries (such as the European Union) as a result of a number of initiatives. These include:

- the development by WHO Regional Office in Kobe, Japan of a tool for addressing health equity in cities: Urban HEART (Urban Health Equity Assessment and Response Tool);[2]
- the final report of the WHO work on social determinants of health led by the Commission on Social Determinants of Health: *Closing the Gap in a Generation: Health Equity through Action on the Social Determinants of Health*.[3]
- the establishment of the European Health Network and the European Portal for Action on Health Inequalities. The EuroHealthNet is a coordinating body funded by the EU for action in Europe, which published *The Right Start to a Healthy Life* in 2012 (Stegeman and Costongs, 2012) , based on tackling the health gradient, associated with a Gradient Evaluation Framework (GEF) (Davies and Sherriff, 2012).

3.2 Research on health inequities

A further support to taking action is the paper by Östlin et al. (2011) 'Priorities for research on equity and health: towards an equity-focused health research agenda' that describes the need for a 'third wave' research programme on health and takes as its focus the importance of a dynamic programme on the social determinants of health and their impacts. In summary, the WHO Commission on the Social Determinants of Health report, which was based on an extensive review of the global evidence, highlighted the need for strengthening research on health equity. Östlin et al. (2011) suggest this requires a 'paradigm shift' to address social, political and economic processes that influence population health and has 'four distinct yet interrelated areas: (1) global factors and processes that affect health equity; (2) structures and processes that differentially affect people's chances to be healthy within a given society; (3) health system factors that affect health equity; and (4) policies and interventions to reduce health inequity'.

To build an active collaboration amongst different disciplines, this type of research demands new strategies from those used in the past, which will include the following (reproduced with some minor changes from Östlin et al., 2011):

- Going beyond behavioural and other individual determinants of illness towards a holistic approach that understands social, economic, political and cultural including health-related determinants and examines 'the intersections amongst different social hierarchies and power structures, such as class and gender, and their cumulative impacts on health status and health inequities'.

- Examining the 'psychosocial' pathways, and power connections across the 'upstream' social determinants or root causes of health inequities in addition to the more traditionally investigated determinants of health inequities, such as risk factors or access to care.
- Treating patterns of health inequity as a 'social reality', requiring social (economic, sociological, political and cultural) explanations that add to the combination and clarification of individual biomedical (health care) processes and outcomes.
- Considering the dynamic (rather than static) nature of equity and inequality in different contexts, introducing a temporal and financial dimension when investigating social structures, public policies and impacts over the life course, and which describes the social institutions and processes that influence the choices, determination and allocation of resources related to health and social care.
- Recognising that certain kinds of evidence, such as results from randomised control trials, may not be relevant to many of the interventions that address social determinants of health; and thus diverse methodologies will be needed that generate both qualitative and quantitative data on the questions being examined.
- Genuinely involving affected populations through carefully designed engagement strategies in developing appropriate research programmes but *prima facie* should move from single risk factor analysis to a broader and more all-inclusive standpoint, involving a multi-factorial analysis.

One of the major issues in health care is how to tackle equity through improved access to health care without 'catastrophic financial burdens' on populations (Östlin et al., 2011). Even in rich countries in the West such as the UK, austerity programmes and cutbacks are exacerbating rather than improving health equity especially, ironically, in relation to those interventions that may have the most benefit in reducing equity gaps or improving the health and health care of excluded groups (i.e. primary and secondary prevention and health promotion). New and updated methodologies are needed, such as benefit-incidence analysis, micro-simulation and long range scenario planning (Östlin et al., 2011). Because funding of health care is a major concern, there is a need to develop better ways to achieve universal health coverage and 'identify sustainable and innovative mechanisms for longer term and predictable forms of global financing' (Östlin et al., 2011).[4]

Similarly there are many factors that affect health equity that are often overlooked but which affect all countries to a greater or lesser extent, such as global warming and climate change (for example, super storms or water shortages), fragility of social structures as a result of warfare, or direct and indirect discrimination against ethnic minorities and socially excluded groups including religious minorities.

3.3 Equity in health care

Health equity can be described in many ways, each of which has differing imperatives for action. Mooney describes seven (Mooney, 1983): equality of expenditure per capita; equality of inputs per capita; equality of input for equal need; equality of access for equal need; equality of utilisation for equal need; equality of marginal met need; and equality of health. The difference between equality of access and of utilisation is in separating concerns for supply and demand (or need). Thus equality of access is about equal opportunity: the question of whether or not the opportunity is exercised is not relevant to equity defined in terms of access. Utilisation on the other hand is a function of both supply and demand. If access, a supply side phenomenon, is equalised, unless demand is the same, utilisation will not be equalised. To these seven we can add equity in ability to benefit, which would strengthen the point about equality of marginal met need. Nonetheless, these seven (or eight or nine) are not mutually exclusive.

A choice needs to be made about the way that equity is exercised and the fundamental values the society wishes to espouse. Evening out the resources to each person may seem equitable but could make things worse if one person requires a health care intervention that is very expensive and another person does not at any stage in their life need more than minor-cost procedures. Similarly, equality of inputs does not do justice to differing need. Equality of ability to benefit requires a prior allocation to those deemed to have a lower ability to benefit which in turn suggests that achieving equity requires two stages: a first stage to level the playing field and a second stage to ensure that everyone is then treated similarly according to their needs.

Inequalities in health describe the differences in health between differing groups independent of their fairness. The term 'inequity' (coined by Margaret Whitehead, and used in WHO documents) refers to differences in health which are not only unnecessary and avoidable but, in addition, are considered unfair and unjust. As Whitehead noted, judgements on which situations are unfair will 'vary from place to place and from time to time', but one benchmark is the degree of choice involved. A useful definition (Whitehead, 1991) is:

> Equity in health implies that ideally everyone should have a fair opportunity to attain their full health potential and, more pragmatically, that no one should be disadvantaged from achieving this potential, if it can be avoided. (Whitehead, 1991)

In other words, using this definition, the aim of government policy on equity and health would not be to eradicate *all* health differences but to reduce or remove those which result from factors that are considered to be both avoidable and unfair, and to ensure that adverse discrimination is outlawed. Consequently, health equity also depends on the values held by individuals, experts, policy-makers or populations, which determine implicitly or explicitly what is fair or unfair. As we saw earlier, values-based practice is an essential component of the toolkit for deciding on health and wellbeing interventions. Agreement and dissensus is common (e.g. gender norms differ in different places) and we may want to agree to differ on some crucial aspect of a health or wellbeing intervention. But equity remains an important goal of any health and wellbeing procedure, whether determined by the NHS or a local authority.

Box 3.1   Definitions of equity found in the literature

- Equity of a decent basic minimum health care to all
  - Equality of a basket of services considered relevant for all in society
- Equity of access for equal need (to appropriate services)
  - Does not ensure equal ability to benefit, or achieve equity in resources or outcomes
  - Equality of access is about equal opportunity: the question of whether or not the opportunity is exercised is not relevant to equity defined in terms of access

- Equity of inputs in relation to need

  o Equal inputs for equal need

- Equity of expenditure or resources available per person

  o Equality of expenditure per capita. Equity of resources does not ensure that resources are spent according to need

- Equity of inputs per person

  o Equality of inputs (resources, people, etc. per capita)

- Equity of utilisation for equal need

  o The difference between equity by access and by utilisation lies in separating matters of supply and demand (or need). Utilisation is a function of both supply and demand. If access, a supply side phenomenon, is equalised, unless demand is the same, utilisation will not be equalised

- Equity of marginal met need

  o This is not based on an equity of starting point for treatment

- Equity of outcomes

  o Outcomes differ according to the person's condition, their illness or disease, and the way the resources are spent. This might be described as equality of health

- Equity in ability to benefit

  o Assuming equity of access, equity in ability requires a fuller programme to deal with social determinants of health and to create a 'level playing field' – bringing everyone to some agreed state of health, if achievable

(based on Mooney, 1983)

'Equity' is thus concerned with creating equal opportunities for health and with bringing health differentials down to the lowest level possible. In our concern for (mental) health and wellbeing we will want to reduce those factors that discriminate on irrelevant grounds whilst carefully ensuring treatment accords to need. But equity is also relevant to wellbeing. We will not achieve maximum wellbeing when, for whatever reason, some individuals and communities are treated less favourably than others. Equity is an essential component of commissioning for wellbeing.

3.4 Commission on the Social Determinants of Health

The Commission on the Social Determinants of Health (WHO, 2008) published a conceptual diagram based on an intermediary report by Solar and Irwin (2007) which is shown in Figure 3.2 (with some minor modifications by the authors). In this they identify three stages: socio-political and economic policies that frame a country's health and wellbeing provisions; the gaps and gradients that flow from the power imbalances created in stage 1; and the material and other circumstances that both create disadvantage but also allow improvements to be made through policy initiatives. The health care system plays its part as a transitional arrangement, mediating some but by no means all the influences on health and wellbeing.

The purpose of the system described is to demonstrate a cyclical approach that draws on the socio-economic context, is influenced by socio-economic gaps and gradients, and affects the health system through various material circumstances, psychosocial factors, behavioural aspects and biological predispositions (Davies and Sherriff, 2011). These in turn influence the socio-economic context. The socio-economic prerequisites are structural determinants: governance, macro-economic policies, social policies and human development opportunities and the culture and values of society. From these we move through a range of socio-economic gaps: as a result of gender or ethnicity discrimination, the implications of deprivation, the effects of education, occupation and, of course, levels of income. All impact on equity; all impact in subtle and not so subtle ways on wellbeing. From this we can see that we must intervene at each stage: review and revise national and international policies (e.g. EU policies that affect the UK); attack historic equity gaps and gradients (what we refer to as prior discriminations); challenge material circumstances and unhealthy behaviours through socio-economic wellbeing interventions; and ensure the health system tackles social determinants of health.

As Popay (2012) has suggested, we must recognise that simply by achieving improved wellbeing outcomes we do not demonstrate either an ethical or sustainable basis for social justice. Only by prioritising human flourishing and capability developments as the aims and means of policy and practice can we release individual and collective capabilities, enable people to exercise their own agency and make best use of scarce resources. In Figure 3.1 we suggest that national policies sometimes deliberately and sometimes inadvertently create vulnerability through policies and practices that encourage marginalisation and exclusion.

Promoting health and wellbeing must not only address health-related behaviours but also the reasons that people behave in the way they do. For example, self-care in depression and diabetes is poorer in deprived communities. If we are to improve diabetes self-care we have to recognise the additional vulnerabilities that are a concomitant of deprivation, not of the persons themselves but the reasons that they came to live in that additionally vulnerable state, often largely as a result of adverse experiences in childhood and structural inequalities. Our interventions will be less successful if we do not address the reasons people live in states of deprivation or vulnerability.

Taking action on health equity is therefore both challenging and complex. Internationally, WHO's *Closing the Gap in a Generation* report (2008) suggests three areas of action: improve daily living conditions; tackle the inequitable distribution of power, money and resources; measure and understand the problem and assess the impact of action. All of these apply to the UK to some degree. 'Inequity in the conditions of daily living is shaped by deeper social structures and processes. The inequity is systematic, produced by social norms, policies and practices, and practices that tolerate or actually promote unfair distribution of and access to power, wealth and other necessary social resources' (WHO, 2008). Health equity should become a marker of government performance and health equity impact assessments should be built into all global, regional and bilateral agreements.

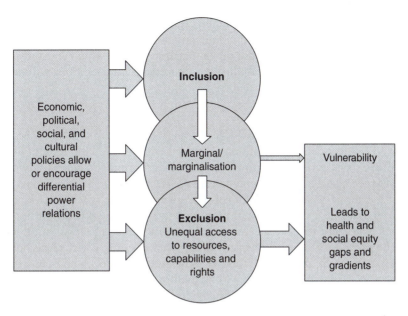

Figure 3.1 Ways in which exclusion and vulnerability are related

Stronger public leadership is needed and gender equity as well as the economic contribution of house work, care work and voluntary work should be recognised.

Equity gaps can be seen clearly when there is a difference between, say, a national average and the average for a defined area. This may be based on ethnicity (health of minority groups in comparison to the majority white population in the UK), gender or any number of factors which define two or more distinct groups. Equity gradients, on the other hand, demand a recognition of social stratification based on education, income, gender or other relevant factors, and differential vulnerability or susceptibility between social groups, or differential consequences of disease, or the role of health events that depend on an individual's socio-economic circumstances (Bornemisza et al., 2010: 81). By stratifying an area into five or seven groups (by one or other of these factors, such as income or deprivation) it is possible to see the gradient effects. Both equity gaps and equity gradients offer slightly different opportunities to tackle improvements in health and wellbeing.

a) Equity from the start

At least 200 million children globally (and probably many more) are not achieving their full potential. This has huge implications for their health and for society at large. Investment in early years provides one of the greatest potentials to reduce health inequities. The Commission on the Social Determinants of Health (CSDH) called for:

- an inter-agency mechanism to be set up to ensure policy coherence for early child development (this was echoed in the Marmot Review of the UK);
- a comprehensive package of quality programmes for all children, mothers and caregivers; and
- the provision of quality compulsory primary and secondary education for all children.

These proposals seem not unreasonable, especially (in the UK context) the first two above. As EuroHealthNet has shown (Stegeman and Costongs, 2012) there is a socio-economic gradient from the most well off to the least well off which demands a proportionate universal approach to child health. The effects of nutrition on child health (especially weight) is an important feature.

b) Social protection throughout life

Everyone needs social protection throughout their lives, as young children, in working life and in old age. People also need security in case of specific shocks, such as illness, disability and loss of income or work. Four out of five people worldwide lack the back-up of basic social security coverage. Extending social protection to all people, within countries and globally, will be a major step towards achieving health equity within a generation. Strengthening universal comprehensive social protection policies and ensuring social protection systems include those who are in precarious work, including informal work and household or care work, is essential. Sadly at the time of writing the British government seems determined to undermine these necessary universal benefits, to reduce the safety net for low income families and force people with disabilities into employment whether suitable or not. Going against the grain of well-researched implications of reduced social protection systems will widen the gap between rich and poor and lead to more distress amongst those less resourced to cope.

c) Universal health care

Access to and utilisation of health care is vital to good and equitable health. Without health care, many of the opportunities for fundamental health improvement are lost. Upwards of 100 million people globally are pushed into poverty each year through catastrophic household health costs. The CSDH called for health care systems to be based on principles of equity, disease prevention and health promotion with universal coverage, focusing on primary health care, regardless of ability to pay. The tautological nature of the CSDH's call for action is evident. Equity is a problem, and the CSDH call is for a health care system based on principles of equity! But this demonstrates the importance of achieving equity in health and social care as a fundamental component of tackling the social determinants of health (and vice versa), and reflects the value of prevention and health promotion as fundamental to an effective and efficient health service.

The CSDH also suggested that the UN adopt health equity as a core global development goal and use a 'social determinants of health' framework to monitor progress. If the resources are used sparingly and wisely then an important contribution may be made. As the CSDH concludes, action on the social determinants of health will be more effective if basic data systems, including vital registration and *routine monitoring of health inequity and the social determinants of health* are put in place so that more effective policies, systems and programmes can be developed. Education and training in equity analysis for relevant professionals is vital.

d) Civil society

Of all the proposals in this area the CSDH suggested that civil society can play an important role in action on the social determinants of health. In the UK this will come from local authorities grasping the opportunities offered by the transfer of public health to local government and the value of Health and Wellbeing Boards. HWBs will have the chance to engage local people in policy development, planning interventions and programme management; evaluation and monitoring of performance; and in developing or implementing an evaluation or monitoring tool for health equity locally relevant to the particular circumstances in the UK.

Possibly the phenomenon most potentially damaging to health and wellbeing is climate change. We have good evidence that the world has already locked in at least a 2 degrees rise in temperature by 2050. Although there is quite a lot of statistical uncertainty it is possible that the rise may be higher, perhaps 3 degrees or more. Whilst the early effects will impact most strongly on developing nations, ultimately it will affect all countries and all parts of the globe. Recent rainfall in the UK is not unprecedented (2012 was the wettest summer for a hundred years, which means it was pretty wet 100 years ago) but the likelihood of further wet weather in the UK is very high. Health is likely to be affected by new vector borne diseases (such as malaria), extreme summer temperatures leading to deaths of older people especially, floods taking their toll on those in vulnerable locations, and loss of food growing regions as drought and desertification continue apace (Friel and Marmot, 2011).

As the average global temperature rises so it will be important to develop more efficient and renewable energy sources, fairer food systems, improved flood defences (particularly in low lying areas) and so on. It may be necessary for the NHS to offer higher levels of food supplements for those in deprived communities, or to focus on alleviating anxieties prompted by floods, or droughts, or food supply problems. Mental health issues are

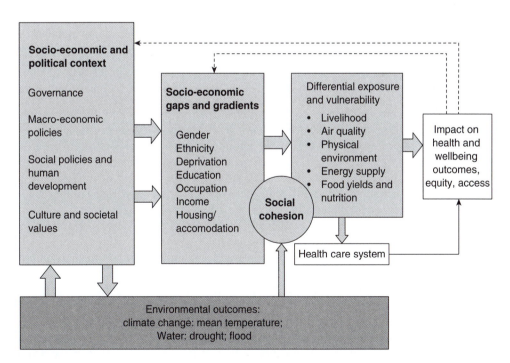

Figure 3.2 Systems diagram of social determinants of health redrawn to reflect the impacts of climate change. Based on a systemic representation of social determinants of health (adapted from Solar and Irwin, 2007, and the report of the WHO/Commission on the Social Determinants of Health, 2008)

probably the most underestimated aspect of climate change and global warming to which the NHS and public health will need to give consideration in the coming five years or so (see, for example, Lyon and Halliday, 2005; Stern, 2006; Grynszpan et al., 2010).

Impacts of climate change can include decreased spending by low-income groups on essential commodities such as adequate, healthy food, security of housing or heating. Mitigating climate change may aggravate poverty alleviation and create greater deprivation; but effective measures to deal with climate change will be a precondition for health equity in years to come (Walpole et al., 2009). But there may also be 'win-wins'. For example, policies to promote safe and accessible use of bicycles could reduce greenhouse gas emissions, reduce air pollution *and* at the same time improve cardiovascular function and mental health.

3.5 Comparability and commensurability

One of the significant problems of tackling health inequalities is the problem of comparability or commensurability between countries. Wilkinson and Pickett have demonstrated in *The Spirit Level* (2009) that income disparity is directly proportional to health equity. The two papers mentioned earlier illustrate this difficulty.[5] Olafsdottir and colleagues' paper on sub-Saharan Africa showed a correlation between state governance of health systems and childhood under-fives health, although it does not demonstrate cross-country and in-country correlations between state action and the disparity of outcomes between socio-demographic quintiles. Conversely Bornemisza and colleagues' paper on fragile states includes some 40 or so countries where the effects of warfare have disrupted many aspects of health and health care, such as cold-chain vaccination systems, as much as the availability of food or clean water. Approximately half of the fragile states are in sub-Saharan Africa reflecting the importance of both micro and macro factors in the challenge of health equity.

EuroHealthNet has promoted the social gradient approach to inequities. The graph in Figure 3.3 is taken from *The Right Start to a Healthy Life*, published in 2012 (Stegeman and Costongs, 2012) by EuroHealthNet, which shows the very steep gradient in life expectancy from professional classes on the left and the unskilled classes on the right.

Similarly the graph in Figure 3.4 taken from the same publication illustrates the subjective health of one and two parent families in four countries. In those countries where inequality is less, then the difference between one and two parent families is less even when the families are materially poorer.

The UK Public Health Outcomes Framework of the Older Peoples' Health and Wellbeing Atlas allows anyone to interrogate the data available. On just three measures we can see the difference between the fifth quintile (most deprived local authorities) and the first quintile (least deprived). Rutland has double the disability-free life expectancy at age 65 – 10.5 years to 5.1 years for males and 11.7 years to 6.3 years for females. But in other areas it is even more stark. Fuel poverty is 29.1% in the worst local authority area compared to just 4.6% in the best; and *excess* winter deaths are a staggering 43.5% in the most deprived against only 6.1% in the least deprived. These gaps (rather than relatively complex multi-factorial gradients where the is no simple uni-directional slope) demonstrate very strongly the way in which those in poorer areas are literally deprived of life, let alone wellbeing.

In Tower Hamlets, for example, mortality from all circulatory diseases for under-75s was more than twice the lowest London borough in 2007 – and that is from a group of challenged areas!

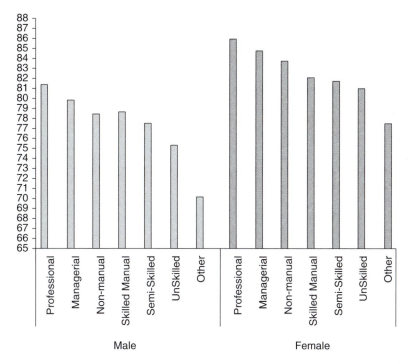

Figure 3.3 Example of socio-economic gradient in Ireland showing life expectancy by social class (taken from Stegeman and Costongs, 2012: 25)

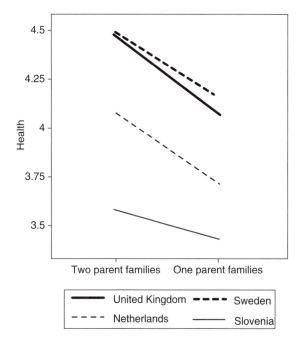

Figure 3.4 Subjective general health in one parent and two parent families (Stegeman and Costongs, 2012: 67)

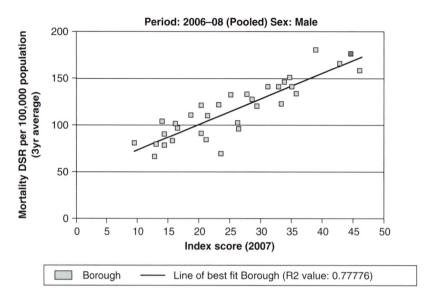

Figure 3.5 Mortality from all circulatory diseases (selected local government areas) showing the twofold difference between boroughs

Similarly, for the disorders which we will consider in more detail below (Chapter 7), CHD and diabetes, the pattern is the same, with inner East London significantly less healthy than the England average (see Figure 3.6). Here we can see the gap without a gradient possibly to confuse the picture. Conversely gradients can very usefully demonstrate other factors that might be involved, especially if income deprivation is not the only or most significant cause.

One approach that has been pioneered by the WHO office in Kobe, Japan is to use outcome indicators and social determinants with a traffic lights (Red/Amber/Green – RAG) scheme to reflect the differing position on each indicator in separate neighbourhoods.

In the example given in Figure 3.8, four disease specific outcomes have concomitant indicators in each of four groups of social determinants, shown here as eight indicators (not described). By measuring the eight indicators across each of the neighbourhoods (in this case, for brevity, six neighbourhoods) a composite score can be obtained for each of the indicators with an average together with upper and lower confidence intervals. This is measured every year throughout the target period until the target is met. (Again, note that for ease of understanding only three years explanatory data are shown in Figure 3.8).

Urban HEART is easy to use – it is a practical approach that is user friendly, comprehensive, inclusive and multi-sectoral, and is operationally feasible and sustainable. Most importantly it makes clear links between evidence and action. Figures 3.7 and 3.8 are taken from the Urban HEART programme paper (WHO, 2005), demonstrating the important factors involved. Areas that may be important for the UK include the four programme areas described in Figure 3.7: infant mortality, diabetes, stroke and chronic obstructive pulmonary disease (COPD), but could include those for which there appears to be useable international comparative data, such as tuberculosis and road traffic accidents. Whilst the specific indicators may not be directly relevant to the UK (e.g. access to clean water or completion of primary education) the process enables different indicators to be incorporated so that the tool is valuable to a UK audience.

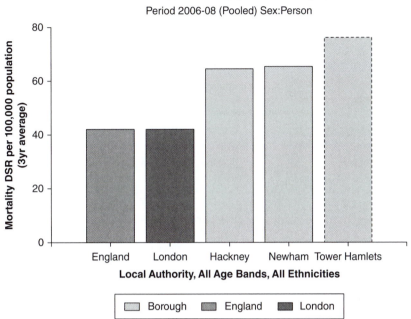

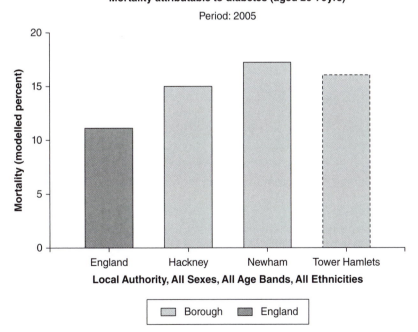

Figure 3.6 Differential mortality for CHD (above) and diabetes (below) with figures for the national picture, London and three London boroughs

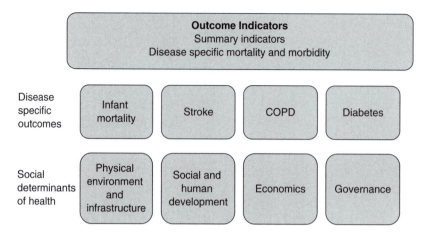

Figure 3.7 A schematic diagram of the Urban HEART tool

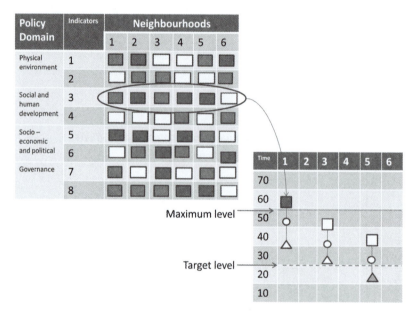

Figure 3.8 A simplified diagram explaining the way that Urban HEART is used

Finally, promising approaches to evaluation of universal interventions have been documented by Milton et al. for WHO in 2010 (see particularly p. 49). They propose that in addition to the usual epidemiological proposals, organisations should adopt other strategies to reduce health inequities, and include:

- innovative ways of exploiting natural policy experiments;
- using logic models and a systems approach;
- cross-national comparative policy analyses;
- resilience approach(es);

- learning from historical analyses;
- the value of case studies.

All of these methods will assist in developing interventions that improve wellbeing and reduce inequities. Whether these are cost-effective is another matter. We will discuss cost-effectiveness and outcome measures in Chapter 11.

3.6 Conclusion

Equity gap and equity gradient analysis can seem complicated and complex, and any use of the techniques described here must recognise some of the barriers to effective action. However, if our actions to improve health and wellbeing do not address the equity problems that may have affected the wellbeing of some patients and service users we will not achieve the necessary changes we envisage. This chapter has made the international case for a national programme to tackle health (and social care) equity as a first step towards health and wellbeing for all. We should proceed with caution but the techniques are effective not only in drawing attention to equity gaps and gradients but in identifying the factors most likely to cause equity differences. Health equity, and developments on the social determinants of health, is a burgeoning field with action being taken by governments and civil society, and commissioners should consider EGA as one component in the process of deciding on priorities for action.

Notes

1 This builds on the success of Sir Michael Marmot and colleagues' work at University College, London University and subsequently the establishment of the UCL Institute of Health Equity in 2011, www.instituteofhealthequity.org.
2 WHO (2005). It is worth noting that although this was developed as an 'urban' health equity tool, the process it adopts could equally be used in suburban or rural settings.
3 WHO (2008). The Commission on Social Determinants of Health (CSDH) was established to support countries address the social factors leading to ill health and inequities, and drew attention to the social determinants of health known to be amongst the worst causes of poor health and inequalities between and within countries.
4 See also papers by Olafsdottir et al., 2011; Bornemisza et al., 2010; Webb et al., 2011 on health equity in fragile states and sub-Saharan Africa where health and social care have been undermined by warfare or civil strife, or by poverty and deprivation.
5 'Health systems performance in sub-Saharan Africa: governance, outcome and equity' (Olafsdottir et al., 2011), and 'Promoting health equity in conflict-affected fragile states' (Bornemisza et al., 2010).

CHAPTER 4

Planning, Commissioning and Evaluating Health and Wellbeing Interventions

This chapter draws on the first three chapters to consider in more depth the role of commissioners and the processes needed to make sensible and effective commissioning decisions.

4.1 Introduction

As we have shown in the earlier chapters, wellbeing is a multi-dimensional concept and the foundation for positive health and effective functioning for an individual and for a community. Thus, responsibility for promoting mental wellbeing extends across all disciplines and government departments and encompasses a concern with social values, culture, economic and social policies, including educational, as well as health policies. In this chapter we set out a framework for commissioning for health and wellbeing, which draws on good practice in commissioning in the context of the current changes to the commissioning landscape, as a consequence of the Health and Social Care Act, 2012. This landscape will evolve and change over the forthcoming years but much of what we are arguing and promoting will still be valid. In particular, there are a number of threshold concepts for commissioners to bear in mind when commissioning for wellbeing whatever the landscape. Much of this book is concerned with exploring these concepts but in this chapter we also provide a brief summary to show how these shape the framework for action.

4.2 The commissioning landscape

The change of government in 2010 signalled a shift towards greater privatisation of health and social care and this may on the face of it sit uneasily with a focus on population wellbeing. However, although this policy direction may be criticised for over-emphasising the responsibility of individuals for their own health, it does potentially incentivise commissioning to prevent poor health. As a consequence of the Health and Social Care Act, which received royal assent in March 2012, new commissioning structures are being developed with the potential of creating an organisational and political space for local innovation.

From 2013, local authorities have a duty to promote the health of their population. They are leading the development of joint strategic needs assessments (JSNA) and joint health and wellbeing strategies, which aim to integrate the local commissioning strategies and ensure a community-wide approach to promoting health and wellbeing.[1] Local authorities are supported by Public Health England, providing national leadership, strategic direction and supporting the overall integration and coordination of the public health system, through four regions and 15 centres.[2] The relocation of public health in local authorities from April 2013 creates an enhanced opportunity to address the social conditions for poor health, whilst responsibility for commissioning health services is now vested in the NHS Commissioning Board and Clinical Commissioning Groups. In early 2012, a Public Health Outcomes Framework was published (DH, 2012a) and this details indicators to meet two broad objectives to:

- increase life expectancy, taking account of health quality as well as length of life;
- reduce differences in life expectancy and healthy life expectancy between communities *through greater improvements in more disadvantaged communities.*

The interventions detailed in subsequent chapters will support commissioners in achieving those indicators that are relevant to improving mental wellbeing through tackling the wider determinants of poor health (e.g. reducing the number of children living in poverty) as well as health promotion (e.g. increasing the proportion of physically active adults), protection and reducing premature mortality (e.g. suicide reduction).

In these new arrangements, the focus on (mental) wellbeing needs to be promoted and the relative lack of awareness of this agenda and its scope addressed. Local actors will be enabled in this task by Health and Wellbeing Boards that are well constituted and engaged with (mental) wellbeing. These HWBs provide a forum of local commissioners 'across the NHS, public health and social care, elected representatives, and representatives of HealthWatch to discuss how to work together to better the health and wellbeing outcomes of the people in their area'.[3] Their aim is to remove some of the barriers to interorganisational collaboration and to engage with local communities in shaping local service provision (see Chapter 5) and to address the wider determinants of health and, over time, to develop an assets-based approach to public health. However, the history of interorganisational collaboration shows that such groups can flounder in the face of the complexity of the necessary interorganisational coordination, compounded by the nature of the task. Health and Wellbeing Boards will be enabled by having a shared vision underpinned by shared values; members with authority to commit their organisations to action; positive leadership and resources; and a focus on values-based commissioning that recognises the importance of engaging communities (Heginbotham, 2012). This will provide a foundation to engage with the demanding task of enabling a focus on prevention alongside service provision. Inevitably, there will be HWBs that make quicker progress on this agenda than others and those that do will have a developed understanding of the task and its inherent challenges with the motivation and capacity to address these. This may well hinge on whether HWBs remain rooted in a traditional 'pathogenic' approach or whether they seize the opportunity to take an assets-based approach to wellbeing, underpinned by 'salutogenesis'.

4.3 Threshold concepts for commissioners

The idea of threshold concepts has been developed for an educational context (Meyer and Land, 2003; 2005) to assist in understanding why some students make more progress than others in getting to grips with 'troublesome knowledge'. It seems to us that if commissioning for wellbeing is to achieve transformational change that we have outlined so far, it similarly requires understanding, analysis and integration of new and complex information in order to formulate a strategic direction. If this process is to be transformative 'it entails a letting go of earlier, comfortable positions and encountering less familiar and sometimes disconcerting new territory' (Meyer and Land, 2003: 54). Commissioning for wellbeing and prevention has rarely pursued the opportunity for transformational change, which would require shifts in current patterns of investment. Rather, commissioning for (mental) wellbeing has typically been characterised by investment in short-term, and thus unsustainable, initiatives, which have not always been built on an understanding of what works, for whom and in what circumstances. However, some interesting initiatives were beginning to emerge as a consequence of place-based commissioning towards the end of the last Labour term in government. Such initiatives were working towards shifting the focus on the response of individual organisations (health, social care, education, police, etc.) to that of a geographic space.

Conceptualising the focus for intervention as a social space (where people live, work, learn, pray, pursue leisure pursuits, etc.) rather than individuals or a service response is an example of a threshold concept. Threshold concepts open up new ways of thinking about a subject that has previously been inaccessible and thus provide a gateway to a new understanding by shifting the perception of an issue and revealing its interrelatedness with other areas of activity or thought (Meyer and Land, 2003). In this book, we discuss a number of threshold concepts that we think have the potential to transform commissioning for wellbeing. Some of these concepts are not new but we think that together they do provide a portal to a different approach to commissioning for wellbeing.

- **Social capital**: the idea that wellbeing is accumulated as a resource, thus revealing the interdependence of individual, family, community and social wellbeing.
- **Health and social inequalities**: the idea that poor health is related to structural inequities, inequalities and disadvantage in access to social and economic resources. Adopting a population perspective ensures that the structural inequalities between different groups within the population, particularly in respect of age, disability, ethnicity, gender, sexual orientation, religion and faith are explicitly recognised and taken into account.
- **Proportionate universalism**: the idea that both universal and targeted interventions are needed and that the intensity of the intervention is proportionate to the level of need.
- **Interdependence of physical and mental health**: the idea that physical and mental wellbeing are intimately connected and thus poor physical health can affect mental health and vice versa.
- **A focus on space:** the idea that the structure and practices deployed in the places where people meet can be a significant factor in their wellbeing and thus provide a focus for intervention.
- **An assets-based approach:** the proposal that greater success in tackling social issues is going to be made by adopting an assets-based approach that reframes the question and builds on

capabilities and not deficits assets (e.g. McLean, 2011). For example, shifting the focus to 'ageing well' from ageing as a negative and problematic experience.

- **Co-production**: the idea that the experiential knowledge and social networks of lay people and communities is as valuable as and complementary to the specific knowledge and technical expertise of health and social care professionals.

Meyer and Land's (2003) paper illustrates the need for commissioners to develop a proper understanding rather than a simple or partial understanding of these key concepts, as people can get stuck part way to a full understanding. In getting to grips with these concepts, health and local authority commissioners, and their partners, can jointly make local decisions about health improvement strategies to suit local circumstances. They enable organisations to focus on improving wellbeing as a central purpose of commissioning rather than an unintended consequence.

4.4 A framework for action

Commissioning, if done well, is much more than simply assessing needs, contracting and then monitoring provision; rather it is a dynamic and iterative process of organisational and service development. Commissioning, framed in this way, is seen as a developmental process and concerned with local learning and this fits well with the introduction of new commissioning structures, which will require time to develop their capacity. However, viewing commissioning as learning, and the process as dynamic and recursive, means that initial commissioning intentions may well be reshaped and adapted as a consequence. Theoretical approaches to implementation typically view this as problematic, emphasising the importance of programme fidelity and suggesting measures for restricting local discretion and thus potentially variations in outcomes. And yet it is the case that contextual factors will play an important role. These factors are not necessarily problematic but open up opportunities for new learning about interventions and programmes (see Chapter 10). Therefore of critical importance is the overall approach to the commissioning task and the need for reflexive commissioning that brings together the value of programme fidelity and the evidence base with a developed understanding of the local context, borne from the active participation of local communities and local people.

> Creating a mentally healthy society entails building up all three facets of the art (creative and effective practice), science (strong research and theory base) and politics (supportive government policies and political processes) of mental health promotion and working across diverse sectors in order to address the upstream determinants of mental health. (Barry and Jenkins, 2007: 1)

Local authorities and health services, together with their partners, have a major role to play in raising the awareness of the factors that influence mental wellbeing and taking practical action through HWBs. This will encompass action to achieve: (a) improvement of physical and social wellbeing; (b) promotion of protective factors; (c) reduction of the impact of risk factors; and (d) creation of supportive environments. This focus on mental wellbeing and population mental health should achieve all the points in Box 4.1 below:

Box 4.1   The factors on which commissioning should focus

- A more explicit focus on commissioning the mental wellbeing component of existing provision.

- Better strategic coordination of exiting activities and aspirations to improve mental wellbeing.

- Commissioning additional activities and increasing upstream investments.

- Using the rapidly developing evidence base on the protective, risk and environmental factors associated with mental wellbeing and of the interventions that can promote mental wellbeing at an individual and social level.

- Understanding and recognising diversity within communities and developing appropriate methods for engagement to determine interventions to strengthen mental wellbeing.

A framework to support Health and Wellbeing Boards in commissioning for wellbeing is provided in Figure 4.1, drawing on Canadian work on commissioning for population health,[4] and is underpinned by the threshold concepts discussed earlier. As this shows, this process is cyclical and thus iterative and will require securing agreement and sign-up from senior leadership within the relevant organisations as well as the key partnership groups, particularly Health and Wellbeing Boards. The HWB and partner organisations will need to identify and invest in capacity to drive this forward.

a) Focus on population wellbeing

A population perspective requires a focus at different levels – social, community and individual – and will involve determining population outcomes for wellbeing, analysing the population health profile and assessing the contribution of local environment. Within this population approach, there is scope for interventions at an individual level, enabling people to take action to promote their own health, and both a universal and targeted approach, i.e. proportionate universalism, as discussed earlier. Whilst addressing structural inequalities, particularly in respect of age, disability, ethnicity, gender, sexual orientation, religion and faith and income, represents a significant challenge, it is compatible with a population focus, as Marmot has shown. Public policy and services, in their development and design, can inadvertently perpetuate inequalities. This understanding needs to be a central strand within the development of local commissioning strategies for population wellbeing so that commissioners remain alert to relevant information and indicators of mental wellbeing for different sections of the local community. This will be enormously helped by engagement and co-production with local people and communities. Focusing on population mental wellbeing has implications for data collection and analysis of demographic data and wellbeing outcomes and there are a range of resources to help with this available on the Network of Public Health Observatories website (see Appendix).

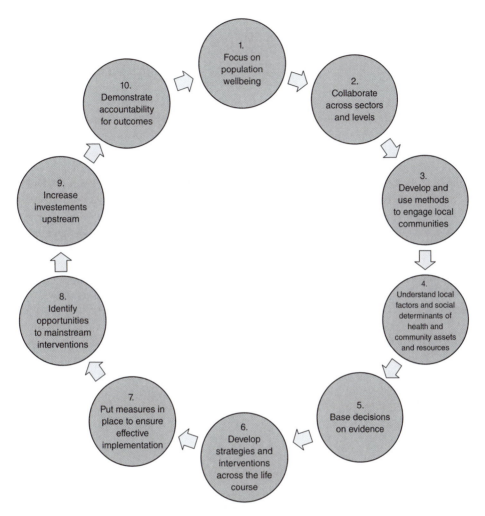

Figure 4.1 Commissioning for population mental wellbeing (adapted from the Public Health Agency of Canada's approach to population health)

b) Collaboration across sectors and levels

The multiple and socio-environmental nature of the factors that shape wellbeing demand that collaboration across sectors is required – involving building partnerships and collaboration across a range of agencies, organisations and community groups within and beyond the health sector – and is a necessary foundation for improving health and wellbeing outcomes. This is recognised in the introduction of HWBs but active engagement across sectors will be needed to promote greater understanding of the concept of positive health and its importance for overall health and quality of life.

Mental health is everyone's business. It is fundamental to all aspects of life – our physical health, our work, our relationships and to achieving our potential. The impact of poor mental health can be devastating for individuals and their families and also has a major impact across the economy. If we are to improve the nation's wellbeing, organisations from across society need to act as catalysts for change in their communities.[5]

To increase the visibility of health promotion at a societal level, a public awareness strategy is also needed to promote greater public and professional understanding of the importance of promoting positive mental health in its own right as a resource for everyday life and societal wellbeing. This means effectively mobilising a public demand for mental health and engaging the participation of the wider community in securing the conditions needed for a mentally healthy society.

On its own this will not be sufficient and the HWB will have a major role in coordinating and driving forward action to improve population mental wellbeing through ensuring this focus is firmly embedded in policy across a range of sectors, particularly education, employment, housing and environment, as well as health and local authority services. Local authorities have a major role to play in creating the environmental and material conditions for wellbeing and through the provision of core services, housing, leisure and education. Commissioning for population wellbeing thus requires a committed multi-agency approach, rooted in integrated commissioning led by the HWBs and the Director of Public Health, reaching out to the Local Area Teams and CCGs, and overseen and driven forward by senior managers, as illustrated in Figure 4.2. This programme should not be seen as an adjunct to existing commissioning, but rather as a fundamental component of a whole system. The mechanisms for this will develop differently across England but in those areas that have a track record of progress in this area, we found the following factors to be present (Newbigging and Heginbotham, 2010):

- committed local leadership;
- capacity and project management expertise in population mental wellbeing to support coordination;
- a task group to coordinate efforts and provide a focus on population mental wellbeing;
- ensuring that members of this task group have delegated authority from their organisations to commit resources;
- setting up mechanisms to work with other key groups that have identifiable responsibilities in this area e.g. Children's Trusts, Sustainable Communities groups;
- identifying opportunities to integrate mental wellbeing within existing strategies;
- identifying actual and potential investment across the partner agencies to progress this agenda.

Achieving impact through the coordinated contribution of the respective partners will be articulated in a strategic direction and implementation plan, which may stand alone or form part of the strategic direction for public health as well as reflected in appropriate policies, e.g. education strategies, healthy working environments, etc. Agreeing a shared vision for population mental wellbeing including aims and impact, a common language and core principles will be an early task. Mapping what strategies and activities are already in place across the whole system and where it would be helpful to align priorities and action to strengthen their impact on mental wellbeing will enable an understanding of the degree of coordination currently in place and that required to achieve maximum impact. A format for this is available in a toolkit that we have previously published (Newbigging and Heginbotham, 2010).

Mental Wellbeing Impact Assessments (MWIAs) have been used to enable a profile of activity and potential areas for development to be identified[6] (National Mental Wellbeing

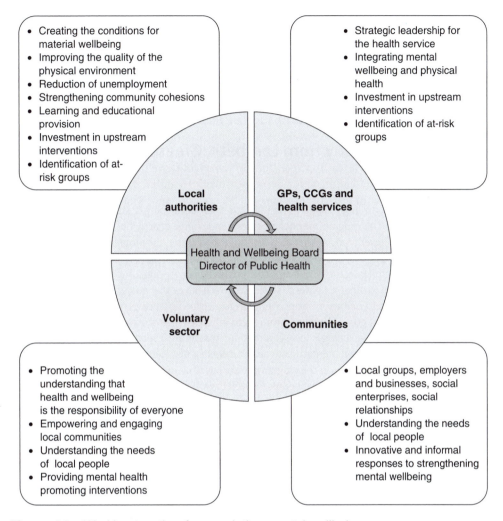

Figure 4.2 Working together for population mental wellbeing

Impact Assessment Collaborative, 2011). Similar to a Health Impact Assessment, the MWIA has a specific focus on mental health and wellbeing and provides a framework for identifying and assessing protective factors for mental wellbeing. An MWIA can be used to assess the potential for a policy, service, programme or project to impact on the mental wellbeing of a population and the process supports the development of indicators to measure impacts.[7] The National MWIA Collaborative have provided a detailed resource to support organisations, including commissioners, to focus on mental wellbeing as an outcome.

A strategy for population mental wellbeing will need to be underpinned by governance structures linked to the HWB to ensure delivery against agreed outcomes. This will include a workforce development programme to ensure that the workforce understands and is equipped to deliver population mental wellbeing. The impact of this strategy on population level mental wellbeing will need to be assessed. However, an over-reliance on strategic intentions may not be sufficient and the energy and commitment of local players to realising this vision will also be necessary. A case study of a strategic approach adopted by Lambeth is provided in Box 4.2 and it is worth noting that, in writing about this development, Smith and Corlett (2011: 23) observed that, as well as the factors identified above, there was a need for 'dogged persistence, and a balance of vision and opportunism'! There is also the need for a long-term view with the first task being to promote the awareness of public mental wellbeing.

Box 4.2   Case Study from Lambeth, Greater London

Lambeth First

Since 2005, Lambeth, an inner London borough, has been developing a strategic approach to public mental health. This programme encompasses a wide range of activities at individual, community and strategic level. Many are initiated and organised within the programme, e.g. through the programme's operational (delivery) group, but many are initiated by others. Activities may be directly focused on improving the wellbeing of the population or specific sub-populations or there may be a contribution to other activities or strategies which have other goals but where there is a need to minimise risks to, or maximise opportunities for, wellbeing (such as redevelopment plans for an area). A particular goal of the programme is to influence mainstream commissioning and service provision so that wellbeing is seen as something that all are responsible for 'producing', i.e. that there is no health without mental health and that there is no wellbeing without mental wellbeing. The content and activities in the programme are based on extensive engagement and this process identified some principles that people wanted to work by and five statements of intent:

- Public spaces and other public assets in Lambeth will be accessible, attractive and safe, and increasingly used by everyone.

- Lambeth will be a vibrant and creative place to live, work and learn.

- Lambeth will be known as a place where people care about each other.

- Lambeth will be an exceptionally cohesive place to live, learn and work.

- Lambeth will be a recognised leader in the provision of sustainable and effective services which enable local people to achieve, maintain and regain mental wellbeing.

Each of these statements had an action plan and was supported by public health capacity. Particular successes include:

- Use of mental wellbeing impact assessments (MWIAs) on policies and services.

- Ten week Spiritual and Pastoral Care course to faith communities on mental wellbeing.

- Developing an approach to measuring wellbeing and producing guidance for use by local services and communities.

- Small grants programme to Voluntary and Community Services (VCS) to encourage work on wellbeing including support with evaluation and training on mental wellbeing.

- A wellbeing network which meets three times a year with monthly wellbeing bulletin to encourage and give permission to others to work on wellbeing.

- Creation of a 'Best Workplace' category of the Lambeth Business Awards.

- Mental Health First Aid and Enhancing Wellbeing training to front line staff in Lambeth.

- Improving mental health literacy through promotion of the five ways to wellbeing message, Mindapples and DIY Happiness.

For more information see: Lambeth First (2009) *Wellbeing and Happiness in Lambeth: The Lambeth Mental Wellbeing Programme*, www.lambethfirst.org.uk/mentalwellbeing (accessed 20 March 2013).

c) Understand local factors and social determinants of health and community assets and resources

Developing the strategy to focus on population mental wellbeing requires information on local conditions, characteristics and trends, with a positive focus on the conditions that promote mental wellbeing as well as risk factors and inequalities, as envisaged in Figure 4.3. This is likely to involve strengthening current JSNA to include information on:

- communities with assets and resources that build good mental health and provide opportunities for strengthening mental wellbeing;
- communities and groups whose mental health and wellbeing are at risk;
- current activity and the gaps and opportunities for investment;
- a population profile and the views of local people and groups as to what matters;
- gaps in equity, the evidence and the priorities for the investment in 'test-bedding' and evaluating new interventions.

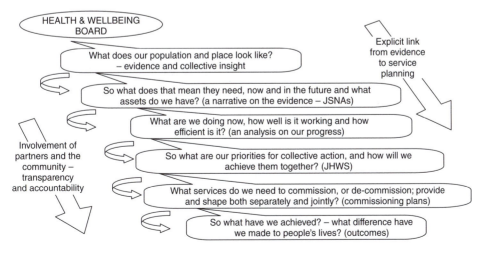

Figure 4.3 Consultation diagram on the way that Health and Wellbeing Boards of local authorities will develop Joint Health and Wellbeing Strategies from the JSNA

By identifying responses to these in a single resource, a JSNA enables local partners to work together and coordinate their planning so that their plans, and investment, are better placed to take action to meet current and future needs. In terms of improving population mental wellbeing it should enable HWBs and their partners to jointly agree the priorities for improving mental wellbeing, having enabled them to start to identify opportunities and avoidable risks in relation to strengthening mental wellbeing.

Box 4.3   Information sources to support the JSNA

Information source	Description	Information relevant to mental wellbeing
Joint Strategic Needs Assessment	From 1 April 2008, local authorities' PCTs have been under a statutory duty to produce a wide ranging and comprehensive JSNA. The role of a JSNA is to provide an evidence base that covers all aspects of the local population including health, mental health, housing, education, deprivation, economy, etc. and should influence all commissioning strategies, service plans and priority setting processes in the local area.	Identification of communities that are mentally healthy and/or have high social capital. Identification of where people with the most and least mental health conditions live. Identification of the groups most at risk of poor mental health. Views of local people on priorities for improving mental wellbeing. What is currently happening and what further opportunities there are to promote mental wellbeing.
Mental Wellbeing Impact Assessment	An improvement method to build the local vision for mental wellbeing and facilitate stakeholder engagement. It provides a method for assessing protective factors and identifying risks to the wellbeing of the local population.	Possible mental wellbeing impacts of service developments, regeneration plans or major policy developments.
Equality analysis	Public sector organisations now have a statutory duty to tackle discrimination and undertake an equality impact assessment in order to narrow the health inequalities that exist in England between people from different ethnic backgrounds, people with disabilities, men and women (including transgendered people), people with different sexual orientations, people in different age groups and people with different religions or beliefs.	Identification of specific issues in relation to particular groups and the potential for disadvantage and discrimination in relation to employment practices, service developments, regeneration plans or major policy developments.

Information source	Description	Information relevant to mental wellbeing
Community assets mapping	This approach starts with the assets in a community and stresses local determination, creativity and innovation with a focus on solutions. The process of engagement and development is a critical part of the process.	Identification of the assets – human, material, financial, entrepreneurial – and other resources in a community that can contribute to building good mental health.
Audit of the likely risks to the wellbeing of local communities	The JSNA should be complemented by a further analysis. This may come from an epidemiological analysis of population changes, such as an ageing population, public health inequalities and health determinants. This data should be disaggregated as far as is possible so that as a minimum it can be considered in terms of gender, age and ethnicity.	Identification of specific risk factors. These could include assessments by the local authority and other agencies of specific problems, e.g. truanting and bullying, increasing unemployment, increasing isolation of older people, levels of violence (particularly domestic violence), levels of crime, environmental challenges, lack of usable public transport, problems of poor housing and other similar factors.

The Association of Public Health Observatories provides information and different data sources to help commissioners to develop their population profile and JSNA. Further information can be found on the North East Public Health Observatory website,[8] including an index of factors that influence wellbeing (Glover et al., 2010) and an atlas of mental wellbeing showing a range of risk and protective factors for mental wellbeing.

In adopting a population perspective the challenge is to ensure that the structural inequalities between different groups within the population, particularly in respect of age, disability, ethnicity, gender, sexual orientation, religion and faith, are explicitly recognised and taken into account. This understanding needs to be a central strand within the development of local commissioning strategies with commissioners alert to relevant information and indicators of mental wellbeing for different sections of the local community. This will be enormously helped by engagement with the public and communities.

One approach that has been adopted in tackling health inequalities is provided by the Institute for Innovation and Improvement, working with the Spearhead group of local authorities (Bentley, 2007). This group comprised one-third of local authorities that had worse health in the early 2000s and where a lot of resources have been diverted to assist in achieving marked improvement. One aspect of this work is its relevance to the role of HWBs as they become established. HWBs will have similar roles in tackling health inequalities and addressing asset-based approaches to public health; by drawing explicitly on the success of the Spearhead experience they might develop strategies that will achieve early improvements.

Figure 4.4 demonstrates a truism about health inequalities as the converse of wellbeing. By engaging communities effectively it will be possible to understand the reason for the behaviours and lifestyles that lead to health inequalities; by bringing frontline health and social care provision to work with communities on the identified health inequalities it will be possible to deliver improved health for individuals; and by aggregating those successes it will be possible to 'square the triangle' and demonstrate a population effect. We will see in Chapter 5 how the community engagement process can be undertaken successfully.

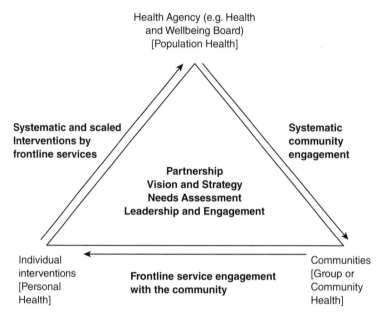

Figure 4.4   Addressing health inequalities

Source: Bentley (2007) for the NHS Institute for Innovation and Improvement

d) Evidence-based decisions

The identification of priorities for action locally will be guided by strategic planning, adopting an evidence-informed approach carried out in consultation with key stakeholders (including members of key target groups for interventions). This entails the following elements:

- a review of current initiatives and a plan for sustaining and scaling up local interventions that have been found to work successfully (i.e. based on evaluation findings);
- systematic use and translation of existing international evidence to guide priority action selection, including the transferability of the evidence into culturally appropriate, feasible and sustainable strategies in the local context;
- balancing innovative local practice with adopting and implementing best practice programmes;
- using assets where these have been shown to be effective.

There are also many emerging and promising interventions and issues or population groups for which the evidence base has not as yet been established. The focus of much evidence has been on the outcomes delivered by specific interventions and further work is needed to understand which programmes work and for whom. Given this, commissioners have a critical role to play in undertaking or commissioning further evaluation of local mental health improvement initiatives to contribute to the evidence base.

Based on the mapping of current activities and the synthesis of evidence provided here, a mapping analysis is a helpful step in identifying potential priorities, and involves three main steps:

- reviewing current activities against the interventions, both universal and targeted across the lifecourse, for which there is strong evidence;
- identifying those initiatives that are working well locally and catalogue the structural, technical and contextual factors that have facilitated their positive effects;
- collating information about the local population and identify whether there are particular groups or communities that are disproportionately disadvantaged by this analysis.

Identifying priorities and making decisions

How evidence is translated into action at a local level is important. A key element of the process is ensuring that the evidence fits the characteristics of the local population and that consideration has been given to how it might be implemented and any necessary adjustments for different segments of the population. The discussion in Chapter 10 explores this further and a crucial element of this is a detailed understanding of the local population stakeholders (including members of key target groups for interventions) through community engagement, as discussed in Chapter 5.

Box 4.4 provides some potential questions for commissioners to assist the process of priority-setting.

Box 4.4   Developing Intervention Programmes

Decide the programme objective

Is the intention to:

- Maximise wellbeing 'gain' overall?
- Target those with the lowest wellbeing?
- Target those requiring additional assistance to benefit from whatever programme is offered?

Determine the target population

Is the intention to:

- Target minority populations with specific deprivations?
- Offer interventions to all members of a community or neighbourhood?
- Target specific population groups, children, women, older people, etc.?

(Continued)

(Continued)

Define the intervention

- What are the core elements of the intervention to which fidelity needs to be maintained to achieve maximum impact?
- What are the important contextual factors that require the intervention to be adopted and what is the potential influence of this on the effectiveness of the intervention?
- What measures have been put in place to ensure that the intervention is relevant and takes account of the diversity of the population (i.e. is it culturally relevant, age appropriate, appropriate for people of different sexual orientations, etc.)?

Achieve maximum health and social gain from the intervention

- What are the main gains and the wider educational, social, economic and community oriented gains to be obtained?

Mainstream the intervention

- How can the intervention be mainstreamed to add value to existing health and social care provision wherever possible?

Develop the most cost-effective solutions

- What is the most cost-effective solution?

There are now many digests of useful information about evidence, with reviews from Foresight, NICE, Social Care Institute for Excellence (SCIE), the Department of Health and independent organisations such as the New Economics Foundation. This evidence base is not comprehensive but is rapidly growing and provides a robust foundation for local health and wellbeing strategies.

To establish a strategic direction it will be necessary to weigh local priorities against the available evidence. This can be done by bringing together the information from the JSNA with the results of the gap analysis to agree which interventions will potentially contribute most to the mental wellbeing of the local population and provide the best investment. The evidence should be triaged as follows, based on national quality assessments:

- **Level 3**: sufficient, well-structured or researched evidence that supports a cost-effective intervention.
- **Level 2**: Some reasonable research information and *prima facie* evidence of effectiveness in practice, although not recorded rigorously. Insufficient information about cost-effectiveness.
- **Level 1**: Insufficient or no research evidence.

Figure 4.5 illustrates a matrix to support decision-making by bringing together the research evidence with local priorities to identify the areas for action by HWBs and local organisations. The matrix ensures that effective interventions are married to local priorities and

Evidence for the intervention	3					
	2					
	1					
		1	2	3	4	5
	Outcomes identified as a local priority					

Key:

Why is this a low priority when the evidence is so strong?

Not a cost-effective investment by definition!

Is this a wise investment given the strength of the evidence?

Or is there a moral or communitarian argument?

High priority but low evidence – are there good anecdotal or 'common sense' reasons for this investment?

Investment should be targeted here if nowhere else.

Figure 4.5 Decision-making matrix: priority levels for interventions are rated on a five point scale from priority level 1 to 5 (where 1 is low and 5 high)[9]

values to promote mental health and wellbeing in ways that are evidence based yet are also culturally relevant and appropriate to local communities.

Thus any intervention is rated by multiplying the ranking of the evidence of cost-effective outcomes (1 to 3) by local priority value (1 to 5). The matrix could then be used to assist in developing the CCG and local authority investment strategies. Evidence-informed practice plays a critical role in demonstrating the success and added value of promoting public mental health and is vital to justifying funding for sustaining initiatives in the longer term. In advancing best practice locally, there is a need to focus efforts and resources on interventions and initiatives that are cost-effective, feasible and sustainable in local settings.

The New Economics Foundation (Robinson and Horwitz, 2012) also suggests government and other organisations should apply the 'ten year test', in other words will the decisions made today come back to haunt us in ten years' time? Nef recommends that the following questions are asked as an antidote to the political imperatives to deliver quick wins:

- How will this policy, this provision, improve lives?
- Will it reduce need or warehouse it, storing up problems for our children?
- How will this investment reduce future liabilities?

We argue in Chapter 6 that the evidence on factors influencing children's future mental wellbeing is strong enough to take concerted action now, although it may be 5 to 15 years until the gains are realised. Similarly, in Chapter 7, we observe that the problems associated with alcohol abuse could have been predicted and some of the current treatment costs averted by preventive action in the 1990s.

e) Impact through partnership

To obtain the full benefits of most interventions it is essential to recognise the holistic nature and multi-sectoral elements of the intervention. For example, successful implementation of universal and targeted support for postnatal depression needs effective coordination and team work between GPs, the primary health care team, health visitors, social workers and secondary mental health care; interventions to promote the wellbeing of elderly people may involve the voluntary sector, primary care, transport and adult education. One of the potential barriers to effective implementation is this multi-factorial and multi-agency nature. Central to these programmes is the role of GPs in supporting individual behaviour change, promoting self-management and providing information, working alongside care managers from social care, voluntary sector agencies and community organisations and other local agencies. As GP commissioning develops, collaboration between social care and GPs to apply proportionate universalism will be invaluable. It will ensure that health messages are delivered universally, without exception; it will also ensure that individuals with specific needs are identified and followed up for targeted intervention.

One agency cannot on its own sustain a programme that relies on several agencies for its effectiveness. However, with multi-agency sign-up, a programme can generate added value through achieving a critical mass of resources focused on the general public as well as at-risk populations and groups. Key decisions will need to be made regarding focusing effort in those areas which are most likely to reap benefits. For example, there is a very robust evidence base concerning the effectiveness of interventions in the early years with families and young children.

f) Balancing investment in universal and targeted interventions

Chapter 2 introduced the concept of proportionate universalism: balancing universal and targeted approaches. Whilst the temptation is to target all the available resources at those most at risk, one unintended consequence of such a strategy is that the programme can become stigmatised, which can then deter those people who might benefit the most from accessing it. However, there are a wide range of universal interventions on offer and introducing mental wellbeing as an element of these would go a considerable way to strengthening public mental wellbeing, for example, in designing urban spaces ensuring there are green spaces, investing in leisure facilities or classes for all, introducing emotional literacy as part of the school curricula – the list is potentially endless! However, universal interventions on their own will not be sufficient because there is a tendency for those who are most resourced to take most advantage of universally available interventions.

The proposal made by Sir Michael Marmot is proportionate universalism and using the example of parenting support, Figure 4.6 illustrates how this balance might be

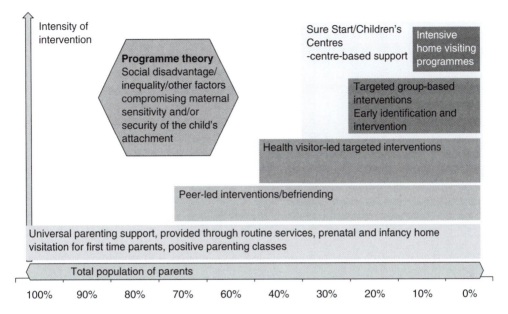

Figure 4.6 Proportionate universalism: an example of parenting support and successively targeted interventions

achieved in practice. The initial universal wellbeing intervention or programme ensures that everyone is covered including those who either do not think it applies to them or would not agree it is needed. In Figure 4.6 we show an example related to parenting skills. The main intervention – the offer of parenting classes – is applied universally: all parents, however well they think they are performing, will get the opportunity to enrol in relevant classes or gain helpful support. From then on the child support opportunities become more and more focused until the most vulnerable are offered a 'sure start' type programme. We will give more attention to this in Chapter 6 when we consider health and wellbeing for children and adolescents.

g) Commissioning interventions across the life course

Commissioning for population health and wellbeing will involve Joint Health and Wellbeing Strategies (JHWS) across the life course, aimed at the general population, those at risk, specific groups as well as interventions to strengthen the social and physical environment. In Table 4.1 we provide examples of commissioning areas, for which there is good evidence, as an illustration of what might be included in local strategies as a starting point. Of course, much more detail will be needed, reflecting the JSNA and community engagement. It is worth noting that although the focus might be on a specific age group, other groups will benefit. This is particularly the case for interventions targeted at adults, where improving their mental wellbeing will have an impact on children and young people if they are parents or older people if they are carers. The following four chapters provide a more detailed discussion on a number of these areas.

Table 4.1 The top ten commissioning priorities (amended from Newbigging and Heginbotham, 2010)

Commissioning area	Specific interventions	Some examples of the impact or outcomes achieved	Implementation aspects and feasibility	References
1. **Promote good parental mental and physical health** to improve early child development and wellbeing, as well as maternal wellbeing.	Universal routine enquiry and targeted treatment for women at risk of depression as part of a package of measures to improve perinatal mental health.	• Improved maternal mental health. • Improved infant and child mental wellbeing. • Reduced maternal postnatal depression. • Improved parental psychological health. • Improved mothers' employment after maternity leave.	Routine enquiry at antenatal clinics. Prenatal programmes with postnatal follow up in the first year after birth are most effective. Interventions with first-time mothers show best effects.	• Independent risk factors for conduct and emotional disorders (Meltzer et al., 2003). • Maternal depression, especially in teenage mothers, leads to behavioural difficulties (Caan and Jenkins, 2009; NICE, 2007; Karoly et al., 2005; Olds, 2002).
2. **Promote good parenting skills** – universal as well as targeted early intervention programmes for common parenting problems and more intensive interventions for high risk families.	Universal access to training programmes: • community-based group programmes; home-based individual programmes, • preschool/early child education programmes, supporting development of home learning environment. Prioritising support for parents from higher risk groups and with children with emotional and behavioural problems.	• Improved parental efficacy and parenting practice. • Improved maternal sensitivity. • Reduced use of NHS, social care, criminal justice and third sector provision. • Build social and emotional resilience from an early age.	Ensure that parenting programmes are universal but where targeting is undertaken match programmes to social context and family circumstances. 10% of parents with children with conduct disorders receive evidence-based parenting programmes. Preschool programmes that combine high quality education with parental support are most effective.	• Group-based parenting programmes have a positive effect on mental health and lead to improved self-esteem (Barlow et al., 2003). • Good parenting skills promote wellbeing and reduce incidence of conduct disorders (Olds, 2002; Cornah, 2003; Bywater et al., 2009). • Social and emotional learning (SEL) programmes improve skills and self-esteem (Payton et al., 2008).

Commissioning area	Specific interventions	Some examples of the impact or outcomes achieved	Implementation aspects and feasibility	References
3. **Build social and emotional resilience of children and young people** through whole school approaches.	Healthy schools; extended schools including supporting families; school-based mental health promotion. School-based SEL programmes achieving pupils' core competencies. Self-management and social skills training. Build financial literacy. Mentoring programmes. Family intervention projects.	• Integrated approach, using universal and targeted interventions in primary school are cost-effective. • Improvement in child social and emotional skills, connection to school and positive social behaviour. • Reduction in conduct problems and emotional distress. • Improved family relationships and improved parental mental health. • Improved self-esteem. • Reduced problem behaviour and conduct disorders including substance misuse. • Improved financial skills and reduced indebtedness. • Reduced antisocial behaviour, reduced domestic violence.	Curriculum should integrate development of social and emotional skills within all subjects, delivered by trained teachers supported by parents. Targeted approaches to children showing early signs of emotional and social difficulties are recommended.	• Peer-led emotional intelligence effective in combatting low self-esteem. Universal school-wide mental health promotion better than classroom-based brief interventions (Bond et al., 2004; Meade and Lamb, 2007; Schachter et al., 2008; Wright et al., 2006).

(Continued)

Table 4.1 (Continued)

Commissioning area	Specific interventions	Some examples of the impact or outcomes achieved	Implementation aspects and feasibility	References
4. Improving working lives: a) support for unemployed, b) creating healthy working environments, c) early recognition and intervention for those with mental health problems, d) supported work for those recovering from mental illness.	Workplace screening for risk of depression followed by CBT where indicated. Early intervention to reduce risks of unemployment through primary care and Job Centres and promote engagement and participation for those who become unemployed. Providing volunteering opportunities. Support NHS, LA and third sector organisations to develop interventions to improve healthy working lives and support occupational health schemes. Stress management interventions tailored to the needs of the employees. Supported work for those recovering from mental illness.	• Increased employment and reduction in lost employment years due to reduced health service and welfare costs. • Costs of programme quickly translate into financial benefits mainly in form of cost savings. • Reduction in health costs of depression and anxiety disorders. • Improved wellbeing due to reduced financial distress impacts on reduced housing stress, etc. • Significant reduction in financial distress. • Reduction in sickness absence. • Significantly improved employment rate for those on a scheme. • Reduction in rehospitalisation. • Reduced time spent in hospital.	Adopt integrated interventions which combine organisational and individual level approaches. Job retention and re-employment programmes which support re-employment and promote the mental health of unemployed people. Supported employment programmes and specialist work schemes are most effective. Reduce mental health stigma and discrimination in the workplace. Support NHS, LA and third sector organisations to develop local interventions to improve healthy working lives, reduce stressors that are beyond the individuals' control.	• Early diagnosis and intervention with employees with depressive symptoms offers good financial return (Hilton, 2005). • Adults who are economically inactive are at increased risk of mental illness (Black, 2008). • Lack of income may lead to increased housing risk and an increased risk of mental disorder (Weich and Lewis, 1998).

Commissioning area	Specific interventions	Some examples of the impact or outcomes achieved	Implementation aspects and feasibility	References
5. Improve the quality of older people's lives through psychosocial interventions which enhance control, prevent isolation and enhance physical activity.	Befriending services (third sector and social care) via social prescribing to target loneliness and social isolation. Group interventions. Falls prevention through social support and education.	• Improved social inclusion. • Effective befriending services would generate significant cost savings. • Improved quality of life. • Reduced A&E attendances and admissions to hospital.	Meaningful group activities with educational and/or support input based on participation of older people. Volunteering and peer support programmes to foster contact between generations. Increasing physical activity in residential care settings and through social prescribing. Ensure staff in leisure centres are appropriately qualified to provide exercise programmes for older people.	• Moderate physical activity improves mental wellbeing (Harvey et al., 2010). • Exercise of moderate intensity has a positive effect on physical and mental wellbeing (NICE, 2008a; NICE 2008b), and reduces anxiety, enhances mood and improves self-esteem (Egan et al., 2008; Etnier et al., 1997). • Volunteering enhances wellbeing more than in younger people (Age Concern and MHF, 2006). • Reduce loneliness and anxiety by providing means to stay active (Lampinen et al., 2006; NICE 2008b).

(Continued)

Table 4.1 (Continued)

Commissioning area	Specific interventions	Some examples of the impact or outcomes achieved	Implementation aspects and feasibility	References
6. **Improving quality of life through increasing opportunities for participation, personal development and problem-solving**	Access to social interventions in primary and community care pathways, e.g. through social prescribing – specifically volunteering, including time banks, exercise, arts and creativity, learning and educational opportunities, green activity. Signposting to welfare advice, particularly employment, provision of support for benefit uptake, debt advice, financial literacy and information and self-help. Debt counselling and advice.	• Self-help groups effective in reducing social isolation/ loneliness and provide meaningful occupation locally, leads to increased quality of life through social interaction and having practical needs met. • Improved mental and physical health. • Increased confidence, sense of community, social cohesion. • Increased levels of social support and caregiver skills. • Reduced demands on primary care and reduced levels of antidepressant prescribing. • Self-management and healthy behaviours. • Increase in benefits through providing access to benefits advice in GP surgeries.	Build collaborative community partnerships based on existing strengths and resources. Use innovative approaches such as social prescribing and mutual volunteering schemes to engage the participation of socially excluded groups. Ensure access to education, learning, arts, leisure, personal development and local support services based on consultation with key stakeholder groups. Place-shaping by LAs to create opportunities for people to come together. Primary care can provide good access to advice services for people in middle and old age.	• Meaningful occupation and physical activity increases overall wellbeing (NICE, 2008b; Casiday et al., 2008). • Time banks generate new social networks and relationships (Friedli et al., 2008). • Adults who are economically inactive are at increased risk of developing a mental disorder (Black, 2008). • Locating welfare advice in general practice increases benefits, particularly disability-related benefits and is an excellent strategy by which primary care organisations can influence their population's health (Greasley and Small, 2005; Abbott and Hobby, 2003).

Commissioning area	Specific interventions	Some examples of the impact or outcomes achieved	Implementation aspects and feasibility	References
7. Implementation of initiatives to prevent, identify and respond to emotional, physical and/or sexual abuse	Building life skills in children and young people including school-based violence prevention programmes including sexual abuse and bullying prevention. Promoting gender equality for women. Reducing the availability and harmful use of alcohol. Victim identification and care and support programmes.	• Reduced levels of mental health problems and physical injuries as a consequence of abuse. • Reduced crime, aggression and violence. • Improved long-term self-management of other conditions.	Multi-component interventions that integrate skills development and training of teachers and parents supported by specialists (see area 1 above). Key role of primary care and the wider health and social services to offer a holistic approach to abuse with an understanding of the contribution of (male) violence and abuse to health and social care problems.	• Physical and sexual violence have direct health consequences and are risk factors for a wide range of long-term health problems including mental health concerns, alcohol abuse, unwanted pregnancy, sexually-transmitted diseases and risky sexual behaviour (Itzen, 2006; Itzen et al., 2008). • Taking a life course approach demonstrates the impact of childhood abuse on lifestyle choices and poor self-management leading to further problems such as diabetes (DH, 2010). Bullying has negative consequences on school health and performance (Bond et al., 2001).

(Continued)

Table 4.1 (Continued)

Commissioning area	Specific interventions	Some examples of the impact or outcomes achieved	Implementation aspects and feasibility	References
8. Integrating physical and mental wellbeing through universal access to lifestyle programmes to reduce smoking alcohol use, substance use and obesity.	Universal access to lifestyle programmes. Targeting higher risk groups, for example people with a mental illness or learning disability, older people and pregnant women. Targeting people with diabetes that are known to be at risk of depression.	• Reduced depression and better self-management of diabetes; reduced dependency on primary care. • Improved physical health and reduction in obesity.	Integrated physical and mental health behaviour change through brief interventions. Opportunistic health promotion interventions for high risk groups through primary care. Skilled staff oriented to respond to the mental health needs of primary care patients.	• Moderate physical activity reduces anxiety, improves mental wellbeing and self-esteem (Hamer and Chida, 2008; Surtees et al., 2008). • People in psychological distress at risk of stroke, acute myocardial infarction, CHD, colon cancer (Etnier et al., 1997; Osborn et al., 2007; Barth et al., 2004).
9. Tackling alcohol and substance abuse, including screening programmes and direct measures with those abusing alcohol.	Screening and brief intervention in primary care. Targeting problem drinking and alcohol abuse through multi-sectoral action (local authority, health, police, education).	• Screening and brief intervention in primary care is highly cost-effective. • Alcohol use reduction has early paybacks and impacts favourably on the NHS reduction in A and E attendances and domestic violence. • Reduce isolation and 'hidden drinking' amongst older people. • Reduction in crime and improved perception of safety.	Multi-sectoral action through multi-agency arrangements between NHS, LAs, police, probation, third sector, etc.	• Effective strategies to reduce alcohol harm require a combination of measures, including police action on anti-social public behaviour and alcohol cost increases (NICE, 2010). • Savings exceed investment costs by 12:1 (Chisholm et al., 2004).

Commissioning area	Specific interventions	Some examples of the impact or outcomes achieved	Implementation aspects and feasibility	References
10. Community empowerment and development interventions that encourage communities to improve physical and social environments, participation and strengthen social networks.	Include encouraging active travel, reducing effects of traffic, functionality of neighbourhood, safe green environments, community arts and culture, volunteering.	Improve wellbeing and quality of life and neighbourhood outcomes: sense of belonging, participation in decision making, wellbeing/ quality of life, satisfaction with place to live.	Use of community empowerment strategies based on the active engagement and participation of local community members. Create awareness of the impact of the social and physical environment on the community and people's mental health.	• Majority of the changes that older people identify as important to their mental wellbeing can be addressed by activities at local level (Age Concern and MHF, 2006). Good cost-effectiveness (Windle et al., 2008).

4.5 Conclusion

In this chapter we have shown how commissioning can be re-geared to focus on mental wellbeing. Key to this is the central role played by Health and Wellbeing Boards to provide leadership across the system and ensure that mental wellbeing becomes everybody's business. We provide an illustration of what could be taken forward by HWBs in Table 4.1, for which some of the detail is developed in subsequent chapters.

Notes

1 Department of Health (2011a) *The New Public Health System: Summary*, http://healthandcare. dh.gov.uk/public-health-system (accessed 9 December 2012).
2 Department of Health (2011b) *Public Health England's Operating Model: Organisational Design*, http://healthandcare.dh.gov.uk/public-health-system (accessed 9 December 2012).
3 www.lambethfirst.org/mentalwellbeing
4 Public Health Agency of Canada, www.phac-aspc.gc.ca/ph-sp/approach-approche/appr-eng. php#key_elements (accessed 10 February 2013).
5 Paul Burstow, Minister for Care Services, 24 July 2012, speaking at the launch of the implementation plan for the No Health Without Mental Health strategy, www.independent.co.uk/news/uk/politics/nick-clegg-sets-out-mental-health-plan-7973046.html (accessed 10 February 2013).
6 www.apho.org.uk/resource/view.aspx?RID=95836 (accessed 13 December 2012).
7 This might be a good point to say more about Friedli et al.'s (2011) approach to MWIA.
8 www.nepho.org.uk/ (accessed 15 February 2013).
9 We are aware that formally public health evidence of the efficacy of an intervention is rated from 1 to 4 where 1 is good and 4 is 'expert opinion, formal consensus'; and that public health rating scheme is from A to D (National Collaborating Center for Methods and Tools (2009); see also Weightman et al., 2005; Rychetnik et al., 2002). We recognise that ours is the 'other way up', so to speak. However, the simplicity of this model is appealing to us and it seems intuitive to give the better evidence a higher score.

CHAPTER 5

Engaging Citizens in Commissioning for Health and Wellbeing

Engaging citizens in different guises – patients, clients, service users, the public and communities – is perhaps the most important aspect of commissioning interventions to improve population health and wellbeing. There are a number of aspects to this, all of which relate to commissioning for wellbeing; engaging individuals in their own care; engaging the public and service users in commissioning decisions; and engaging communities to tackle health and social inequalities, often referred to as community engagement. In this chapter we explore engagement, its purpose, the foundations for good practice and the importance of understanding different values, as expressed in the emphasis given to specific outcomes or processes, that engagement can illuminate. This is not a how-to guide as these are available elsewhere; rather we are concerned to tease out some of the fundamental aspects of citizen engagement in commissioning.

5.1 Introduction

Engaging patients and the public in the commission and provision of services is a statutory requirement of the Health and Social Care Act (2012), with a duty on councils to inform, consult and involve stakeholders having previously been introduced in April 2009. The emphasis on working together to involve citizens in decisions about their local area is strengthened in the current focus on localism. Participatory approaches that engage and build capacity within communities and groups are therefore central to promoting mental wellbeing. The importance of engagement, in its various guises, has been recognised for more than 20 years and consequently there is much for commissioners to build on in terms of good practice in engagement in commissioning, provision and research (Aked et al., 2010; Coulter, 2009; NHS Confederation, 2012a; Nesta, 2012; National Coordinating Centre for Public Engagement,[1] Involve[2]), including toolkits developed by local organisations and widely available on the internet.[3] From the perspective of commissioners, community members and groups, voluntary organisations, charities and social enterprises can make an invaluable contribution to identifying needs, gaps in provision, community assets and significant contextual factors that may enhance or place mental wellbeing at risk. However, there is a shift from top-down conceptions of engagement to recognition of both the value and necessity of working with citizens to co-design and co-produce services, which will challenge established understandings of need, desired outcomes and therefore potential solutions. Alongside this, there is an increased appreciation of the role that people play in their own health and wellbeing, although without a developed understanding of this as a consequence of engaging patients, service users, the public and communities in developing these approaches, there is a risk that they may be misguided, unacceptable and ignored.

Community engagement is a central strand of adopting a population focus because it broadens the scope from thinking about individuals to thinking about communities, whether that is people in a geographic location, people with similar interests or a shared identity. The term is used in different ways and often adopted as a generic term for a variety of methods and models of involving patients, service users and the public in health and social care. It has also come to refer to the involvement of communities and groups, specifically those that are disadvantaged or marginalised, in tackling inequalities (Popay, 2006). In this chapter we focus on community engagement in both senses, to maximise the potential impact on commissioning and thereby potential wellbeing outcomes.

5.2 Purpose of engagement

One of the consistent messages from summaries of good practice of public involvement and community engagement is to establish clarity about the purpose of engagement and for this to be meaningful and fruitful; this goes well beyond the recognition that engagement has become a statutory requirement. This raises an interesting question about why people want to engage in commissioning. Our experience of engagement, particularly community engagement and service user involvement activities, spanning more than two decades, is that people want to make a difference to other people's lives based on their personal experiences, directly or indirectly, of inequalities and injustice. Using a life story approach to understand pathways through participation, Brodie et al. (2011) identify four overarching motivations for involvement:

- Values and beliefs: a set of beliefs and principles, both secular and faith-driven, that people express through involvement.
- Issue: a specific issue that drives people to become involved.
- Interest: a general interest or curiosity that leads people to become involved.
- Skills: a set of skills or experience that people feel could be put to good use through involvement.

Reflecting on individual and community motivations for becoming involved underlines the reality that commissioners and citizens will have different perspectives on the purpose of engagement, reflecting different values and understandings about what is important in terms of change, the outcomes and the process by which these can be achieved. This indicates the need for the purpose, and process, of engagement to be negotiated as well as exploring differences in values, as we discuss later. Where there is limited scope for this, openness and transparency about the purpose of involvement is needed as well as a critical reappraisal of the constraints. In general, the purposes of engagement in commissioning for health and wellbeing will cover:

- understanding what wellbeing means for diverse communities and groups and the specific protective and risk factors;
- understanding community assets and gaps;
- a clearer understanding of individual and community needs, and in particular the diversity of needs, and the potential ways in which these can be met through individual and community resources, and voluntary sector and statutory services;
- raising awareness of the benefits of lifestyle changes and developing strategies for engaging individuals and families in self-management;
- personalising supports and resources;
- addressing inequalities and discrimination, enabling people to realise their potential;
- better informed decision-making and policy development;
- more effective targeting of policy and resources.

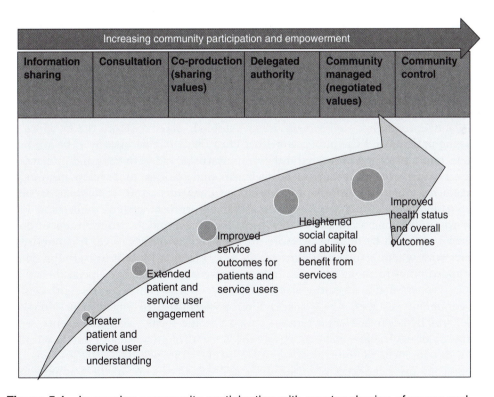

Figure 5.1   Increasing community participation with greater sharing of power and responsibility (Adapted from Popay, 2006)

Therefore, engagement if done well has the potential to broaden the range of options under consideration, to generate really novel solutions and to facilitate social inclusion, solidarity and system growth.[4] The process of engagement is as important as the outcome and indeed they are inter-related with the process contributing to improving individual and community wellbeing. Reference is often made to Arnstein's (1969) 'ladder of participation' to differentiate methods, based on the distribution of power between statutory authorities and citizens. As Arnstein argues, there are a range of initiatives used under the guise of participation but which in reality may require little in the way of engagement (e.g. information-sharing) or may be tokenistic (consultation). In Figure 5.1 (adapted from Professor Jennie Popay's work), it is suggested that outcomes improve dramatically as involvement moves along a scale from passive information provision to active managerial control of services or care provision.

The scope for achieving benefits from genuine engagement and control by communities and groups is clearly within the gift of commissioners. Unfortunately community engagement has not always been done well everywhere. Many differing ways have been suggested, as shown in Box 5.1 below. Community engagement incorporates direct service user engagement (or some form of facilitated user engagement with advocacy by, with and on behalf of service users); public involvement, which has been popular as public and patient involvement, sometimes done more in the breach than in reality; community engagement, per se, where a range of methodologies have been developed; and co-production as a shared activity based on mutuality and a conception of citizens as active agents not passive recipients (Williams et al., 1999).

5.3 Types of engagement

Engaging patients and the public is neither cheap nor is it necessarily easy. We need ways to tap into communities' natural social networks and pathways and understand values and aspirations, obstacles as well as opportunities to develop meaningful engagement. Obtaining information about what matters to an individual or small group of individuals in a street, or with a defined problem such as diabetes, is relatively easy; obtaining a composite set of values and aspirations from groups of users across an area will be immensely more difficult and more expensive. It is important to start with where people are, particularly in engaging seldom heard groups. There are opportunities to engage people (and to intervene) where people spend their time, especially where that is a healthy place – schools, colleges, sports centres, faith centres and community centres. These spaces offer possibilities for engagement alongside more formally organised opportunities with a specific focus – listening events, work groups, co-design events, etc. – alongside the central role that HealthWatch will play in the development of joint health and wellbeing strategies (DH, 2012b). Box 5.1 distinguishes different types of engagement and describes some of the methods used. And as can be seen these have potentially different purposes and use various methods to achieve these.

Box 5.1 Different types of citizen engagement and methods used

Service-user involvement	Public involvement	Community engagement	Co-production
Description			
• Direct involvement of people with experience as experts in a variety of ways – training, research, etc. • Individual involvement in treatment and decision-making	• Involving people as citizens in key, often 'hard' decisions • In commissioning and/or service development and/or evaluation • Collective • Representational	• Involving communities, particularly disadvantaged groups, in a range of activities to improve health and/or reduce inequalities • Process as important as outcome – emphasis on capacity building	• An equal partnership between commissioners and communities/ service users so that activities are co-produced • Based on principle of mutuality, building on what people can do and engaging a range of networks outside services
Types/models			
• Person-centred planning • Feedback/ complaints • Individual/collective advocacy • Service user innovation • Co-design – using the experience of service users to design services with staff • Service provision	• Elected representatives • Consultation exercises • Surveys • Citizen's panels and juries • HealthWatch	• Neighbourhood committees • Community forums • Community champions • Community capacity building • Service provision	• Co-inquiry • Co-design • Co-production of services • Service provision

Four levels can be suggested for action and improved understanding as a basis for commissioning interventions (Heginbotham, 2012). These are illustrated in Table 5.1. Each of the four levels demands a different engagement or involvement process based on two main factors:

- the way in which the engagement processes can be undertaken; and
- the outcomes that the level can deal with adequately.

Table 5.1 Four levels of engagement

Level	Examples of focus	Examples of interventions
Population	Outcomes-led commissioning recognising epidemiological research that informs universal interventions (e.g. such as universal parenting schemes)	Identify and address environmental and social factors and their relationship to outcomes. Support self-management and empowerment and ensure links to appropriate resources. Identify those that need targeted resources
Community	People in a local authority area or community with specific issue demands (e.g. thalassemia in UK families of Greek extraction where these cluster in a local authority area)	Understand assets, concerns and specific challenges. Outreach to understand non-engagement. Encourage advocacy to promote the development of appropriate strategies. Develop and target resources appropriately. Raise awareness of primary prevention strategies
Group	Groups of people with similar or related conditions (e.g. those with Type 2 diabetes, or who are severely obese; or people of South Asian descent with chronic hypertension) or facing similar psychosocial hazards (e.g. disabled people and people with long-term conditions at risk of poverty, unemployment and depression)	As above
Individual	People using a range of services, who may have a specific condition or require specific support	Personalising health improvement strategies and access to appropriate resources. Improve skills of front-line staff and primary care professionals

Engagement is essential for personalisation of interventions for wellbeing and health inequalities. But engagement is also essential for understanding the values of the community. Values matter as much as attitudes; values provide a longer lasting programme on which to draw as they express a deeper core of a community's feelings. Within a process of engagement that considers a specific intervention or set of interventions for, say, alcohol abuse, values offer a basis for making decisions on many subject areas. One example that we will see in more detail in Chapter 8 concerns diabetes. Table 5.1 illustrates a comprehensive approach to community engagement that targets patients and service users, engages professional staff and encourages self-management with appropriate support and care in the context of a public health awareness campaign, understanding the opportunities and constraints faced by specific groups and communities as well as the population level risk and protective factors. Doing all these things simultaneously offers the greatest opportunity to improve health and wellbeing.

5.4 Good practice in engagement

Community engagement (CE) has a number of methodological problems (NICE, 2008c). There is no single definition of either 'community' or 'engagement'; no two definitions are the same. More importantly, CE has rarely been the subject of research which has focused on the outcomes of the process rather than the process itself. Much CE is apparently not cost-effective or the cost-effectiveness calculations can be over-turned fairly easily by slight changes to certain assumptions. On the other hand the lack of an engaged community has led to services that are less good or effective. This is true of many CE approaches from collaborative methodology, to health trainers and citizens' juries (NICE, 2008c: 16). In practice, however, there are four important interlocking themes to maximise success in CE: setting up the projects properly in the first place; establishing an appropriate organisation; systems that encourage and support CE; and evaluation of the project.

Some places have seen the benefits of engagement that goes well beyond tokenism; but too many Primary Care Trusts (PCTs) and local authorities in the recent past have been only too happy to do a handful of focus groups that just about meet the promises they made or the requirements of the service. CCGs and the NCB, and the HWBs of local authorities now have an opportunity to do this properly, genuinely to understand the views of local people, their values and aspirations, what they will stand for and what will put off them engaging with commissioning.

Community engagement must be a genuine attempt to understand the needs of the community in a way that engages the majority within the community. This means engaging ordinary citizens as well as 'community leaders' – councillors, imams, priests, GPs and so on – those who are considered to 'speak for' the community. To achieve this goal, however, requires a new understanding of the community, for example the ethnic mix, languages spoken, religious affiliation and how it is structured, as well as incentives and rewards for taking part. Many people will not want to become involved for the sake of it.

Box 5.2   Foundations for good practice in community engagement

- Supporting capacity for engagement.
- Being clear about the purpose – to provide information, give feedback, advise, generate innovative solutions, make decisions, etc.
- Involvement clearly valued and demonstrated by actions – reimbursing travel and expenses, paying a fee for contribution, providing refreshments.
- Transparency and honesty – establishing any limits to involvement, i.e. who will be making the decisions.
- Processes and mechanisms in place to support people to participate on an equal basis, which might mean training and development for HWBs.
- Range of methods, avoiding an over-reliance on representative structures with specific efforts to reach out to those whose voice is least heard.
- Demonstrate the difference that involvement and engagement have made.

Personalisation of health and social care demands a reappraisal of the role of engagement. Only a comprehensive approach can ensure that service user and community inputs are 'drawn in systematically', that tokenism is avoided as much as possible and that a continuing dialogue is developed and sustained. Tokenism is too easy a trap to fall into, especially the form of tokenism that accepts a small number of rather badly designed focus groups as the sum total of the engagement process. Frequently health commissioners have been guilty of trying to cut corners, reducing the scope of the project, because of time or financial constraints, only to regret it later. Setting artificial deadlines and boundaries is usually counter-productive as the results of the exercise are likely to influence health and wellbeing interventions for some years to come.

A good engagement process will ensure that all segments of the community are drawn in using appropriate and culturally relevant approaches, relevant minority languages, in settings valued or acceptable to the community, and in ways that will not cause offence to the people involved. Those people that are 'seldom seen, seldom heard or seldom listened to' should be considered and efforts made to meet with them and if necessary special assistance should be offered for them to come forward. In this way commissioners can develop a much fuller and rounder picture of those for whom interventions will be commissioned. There is little point in commissioning an intervention for a community that ignores the offer or turns its back for a good reason.

a) Recognition and engagement of minority groups

Health and social care organisations need to understand the values and culture that underpin and contextualise minority values, whether those are of black and minority ethnic communities, disabled people, the values of gay and lesbian groups, and so on. These have and will continue to change so that no previous research or values statement is a reliable guide to how individuals or communities think at present. Many PCTs have had a narrow view of minority communities' values. Although black groups may have many values that are the same or similar to white or other minority ethnic groups, there will be some important differences that should be addressed. Two critical issues need to be recognised. First, the values and approaches of some people, such as those of south Asian heritage, may have been shaped largely by differences in faith and religion and their inherent understandings of the way the society is structured; and second, issues of race and ethnicity are often complicated by or overshadowed by income deprivation, educational attainment or lack of work opportunities, largely as a result of discrimination.

Talking about minority communities as focused on ethnicity misses a powerful point about the range, scope and nature of minorities. The Equalities Act 2010 sets out eight categories on which discrimination is outlawed: age, gender, ethnicity, sexual orientation, faith or religion, disability, carer status and class or deprivation. Ensuring that the values of all those groups and communities are considered is a challenge for CCGs and HWBs. Whilst we can know some of their values some of the time, we cannot, without careful and *frequent* analysis, understand the implications. But this misses a critical point about values.

Working with black groups or any other minority group demands commitment to ensuring the research benefits the group directly, not the researcher or funding body. This can be achieved by working with communities in new and exacting ways. Training volunteer researchers within communities; obtaining research funding that is free of bias and control; working in those communities with staff who have a similar ethnicity, or gender, or language. One project on the reasons that south Asian heritage mothers did not use statutory services in Blackburn utilised two women members of staff, both Muslim, who spoke Urdu fluently. Another project with the gay and lesbian community in Manchester recognised the strongly held values of equality and acceptance, recognition and redistribution, which underwrote the project.

Recognition is an important value in commissioning (Fraser and Honneth, 1997). Recognising ethnicity, or gender, or faith places a responsibility on the commissioner to redistribute resources to meet their needs in proportion to their recognised importance. That may mean existing services being cut or curtailed with the attendant opposition that will inevitably occur. That is better than perpetuating a system that is at once unfair and likely to (re-)create further inequality. By listening to the group or community it will be possible, slowly at first and then with increasing speed and emphasis, to develop a portfolio of services that represent a values-based reflection of the needs of the whole community.

Engaging all sections of the community, especially minority groups, is an essential characteristic of values-based commissioning. How this is done will depend on the nature of the group and the questions to be asked. By working with all cultures and shades of opinion commissioners will be able to balance competing demands more reasonably and address the discriminations felt and expressed by minority communities.

b) Values-based commissioning

The key point is that we are concerned with values, not with the decisions on resources or organisation, important as those are; nor with the developments of interventions for wellbeing. The aim of values-based commissioning is to establish a CE programme that learns from the service users, from them alone or in dialogue with professional staff and others. In its most robust form we need a strong process that recognises the importance of a wider and deeper understanding of values that will stand the practice in good stead. Many commissioners in the past have developed at best a weak system that goes only so far in detailing the values of the group, community or population, and in doing so cannot really understand the deeper values and inherent beliefs of the group or community.

Understanding values is not a process that has been attempted frequently. 'Standard', somewhat limited and traditional CE processes have been used but none of these has attempted to mine the fundamental values that apply to the decisions taken. Values can be ascertained using all the standard mechanisms amended or adjusted to elicit values rather than other objectives. For example, a citizens' jury can be used to decide on the balance between competing health priorities but may also be used explicitly to identify the values that the members of the jury bring to the decisions. Similarly, focus groups may be used to obtain views about the status of different health or social care initiatives but may also be used carefully to understand the values that the members bring (Heginbotham, 2012).

The range of approaches described in Box 5.1 can be used to generate values but were not set up with that in mind. Although many approaches have been used a number of factors prevent them being effective. These include:

- the culture and attitude of statutory agencies;
- the dominance of professional elites and their cultures;
- competing priorities within the statutory agencies;
- skills, abilities and capabilities of staff;
- capacity and willingness of patients, service users, clients, carers and the public. (modified from Pickin et al., 2002, quoted in NICE, 2008c)

In practice, CE and the involvement of patients, service users and carers in determining values is not easy. It offers the opportunity to have a meaningful and much deeper conversation between service users and professional commissioners (GPs, nurses, managers, etc.) and as such is and becomes ever more rewarding. As Whitehead and Popay (2010) have shown there is a welcome improvement in service, social capital, empowerment and health outcomes in moving from informing, through consultation and co-production, towards delegated power and community control. By engaging communities, health and social care staff are likely to make much better decisions on what will work, understand the social return on investment and will thus be more cost-effective as commissioners.

Delegating power and community control may not be possible or desirable in all cases, but in some services where personal budgets (in health or social care) are available, improved outcomes are achievable. Any attempt to commission the best care and support from health and social care within the resources available to meet the needs, wishes, aspirations and (especially) the values of service users, can be achieved by improving the understanding of values and their use through a process of greater community control. Not only do health outcomes improve but a range of service and intermediate social outcomes improve also (see Figure 5.1).

Values-based CE demands different processes from those attempts to define the objectives of service development or health improvement. Whilst JSNA, and associated assets assessment is a critical (and values-based) programme, it does not help directly in determining the values that need to be considered for commissioning. JSNA depends on but does not explicate values (Heginbotham, 2012). Differing approaches to CE are underpinned by differing values systems and it is thus necessary to clarify what we want to know. We need to distinguish community values, but we also need a process for recognising values that are *not* acceptable, such as racist or sexist values. Values can include judgements that most right thinking people will not accept; but similarly we must not exclude values just because we (in our statutory roles) find them uncomfortable.

Certain elements of the NICE Guidelines are worth noting. For example, action in relation to engaging communities suggests that those running a project should:

- encourage local people to help identify priorities;
- consider diversity training and raise cultural awareness;
- encourage all communities to express their opinions (regardless about whether they disagree with national, regional or local policy);
- give weight to the views of local people when decisions affecting them are taken;
- manage conflict between and within communities, and the agencies that serve them.

What these recommendations miss, from a values-based perspective, is just that, the values of the community. Priorities come from deeply held values and diversity is a significant source of values. 'Opinion' should be values-based or it becomes simply self-serving or discriminatory: giving weight to local people is acceptable as long as it can be justified on a values basis – not slavishly but reasonably, frankly and thoughtfully. Conflict can only be managed if the tenth principle of values-based practice is observed – dissensus (Heginbotham, 2012). Communities, the NCB, HWBs, CCGs and local people, should accept the notion of dissensus – being able to agree to differ, honestly, respectfully, appropriately, magnanimously. In the NICE Guidelines there is a call to identify how power is distributed and to 'negotiate and agree ... how power should be shared and distributed'. Making all parties aware of the importance of power within community involvement and in particular the importance of diversity and difference is another important step. A paper written some time ago (Barker and Peck, 1987) described 'power in strange places'; but that is what may need to be fostered to enable communities actively to take responsibility and control.

Engagement priorities establish the scope and depth of the engagement process. It is essential for HWBs, area teams of the NCB, CCGs and other agencies to cooperate in order to understand fully the short, medium- and long-term goals of the community and of professional staff, and why those differ. The third sector has a valuable strategic and operational role to play especially to get to the 'seldom seen, seldom heard, seldom listened to' groups who are least likely to access health resources or organisational arrangements. Perhaps most importantly, health and social care agencies need to connect engagement processes to outcomes. Here values are also important. In many cases outcomes are not readily evaluated as biological marker improvements but are qualitative measures of improvements in general functioning or subjective assessments of 'betterness'. That is certainly true of wellbeing. Improved health and wellbeing requires social marketing of prevention and health promotion; inter-sectoral partnerships for case-finding and lifestyle change initiatives using a proportionate universalism template; removing barriers and improving access to care; and supporting self-management and improving motivation. The last is particularly important as we will see in Chapter 8 on self-management in diabetes.

What matters, however, is how we build on this advice to develop a values-based system. The evidence is sketchy but suggests that we need to have a composite process that draws from the four levels and examines the way that values are used by different groups. Black and minority ethnic groups will have differing values related to their ethnicity, recent country of origin, culture, faith and religion and their present place of residence. Some of their values will be common to the majority, some will be very different. Similarly older people, or lesbian and gay or disabled people, will have some similar and some different values. Some of these values may seem odd to another group, for example professional staff of services, but careful assessment will demonstrate how they have arisen and why they matter. No individual's values are better than anyone else's. They differ, and that difference must be used to throw light on the way that health and social care is managed.

The four levels of involvement in values-based practice need to be brought together into an effective programme that builds on the right mix of different components. To be genuinely effective requires that commissioners consider the values that they will need for the decisions that they have to take. If a 'weak' system is used it will be easier initially and much harder later to get patients and service users to engage meaningfully. Conversely, using a 'strong' system will take time at the beginning but save time later.

5.5 Developing an engagement strategy

When it is decided to develop an engagement strategy, there are a number of important questions to address:

- Which level are we concerned to tackle?
- Which issue or issues do we want to understand?
- What is the policy on implementing personalisation properly?
- How much money or other resources is available?
- When do we have to make a decision on the resource allocation question?
- What interventions or services will be affected?

As we seek the answers to these questions we can see the need for a composite and comprehensive policy that achieves the most critical objective: to understand the values and the interplay of values of individuals, of the group, or community or population that we have targeted. In Chapter 4 we described the health inequalities intervention triangle that identified the role of engagement in establishing targets for the process. (See Figure 4.4 above).

The right-hand side shows the role of a systematic CE process in understanding the way that population health can be and is influenced by the roles and attitudes of communities and groups within those communities. Understanding their motivations will assist in devising interventions that will work for that community; understanding why they continue to enact poor health behaviours will offer pointers to ways in which they can be changed, and understanding the way that assets can be mobilised will demonstrate the way in which assets can modify the deficits targets, which will improve the inequalities (see Figure 1.5, which shows the deficits and assets models side by side).

5.6 Localism

Adding to the potential confusion, the Localism Act 2011 brings a new layer of complexity to the consultation process placed on local authorities. One recent consultation exercise by Department of Communities and Local Government (DCLG) on the 'Community Right to Challenge' was about the opportunity for community and voluntary bodies, parish councils and authority employees to bid to take over the running of local authority services. Many local authorities recognise the role that some groups can play in designing, commissioning and delivering local services, providing new ideas, a deeper and often better understanding of service users' needs, and offering good value for taxpayers' money. The Localism Act 2011 gave these groups the chance to bring proposals about running a service to the local council and required it to give them proper consideration. How this will impact on health and wellbeing is unclear, although it is fascinating that it was introduced at the same time that CCGs were being established. Undoubtedly it has strengthened values-based commissioning, and the values of communities and local groups have taken on a new importance.

The 'Community Right to Challenge' includes opportunities for voluntary groups to express an interest in running council services, even if they presently make a surplus.

Localism must serve more than those with the loudest voices, the most strident views and the deepest pockets. Overall, a balance will need to be struck by commissioners, especially CCGs, between driving power down to communities and retaining the facility to deliver strategic national infrastructure such as new nuclear power stations. By and large, local government staff and others of a statist mindset need to move beyond the 'state' and find ways to engage broader sections of society in shaping their neighbourhoods and empowering people.

What is unclear is the extent to which the Localism Act will be used to develop genuinely robust consultation and alternative service elements for public health and HWBs, especially in relation to housing. Local councils may run with new and quite different interpretations of what consultation means, and assume that the purpose of localism 'to create a range of interpretations. A Cooperative Councils Network (launched in Rochdale on 15 July 2011), set up to tap into the mutualism and cooperative systems that run deep in the history of the left in the UK (Reed, 2011), draws inspiration from the values of fairness, accountability and responsibility (compare Whitehead, 1991 on equity in health). It offers a population slant on values, and a way to understanding how broad values shape services, within which individual and group values can operate.

Box 5.3 Community engagement and community cohesion

While community forums in Newham were seen to work well for some people they were perceived as working less well for others. Through its Community Participation Unit, Newham Council has therefore shifted its focus from engagement structures to engagement via activities, developing a varied programme of community events which engage diverse groups of people in a range of different ways. 'It's all going to be about doing now,' officers explained. These activities have included reading days in the library and community festivals – with the aim of getting people along and then engaging them in discussion on other issues (consulting them on priorities using questionnaires or other more creative engagement techniques when they are attending these community events). There was a positive appreciation of this approach. However, concerns were also raised about capacity-building and future sustainability.

Source: Blake W. et al. (2008: 62). *Community Engagement and Community Cohesion*. York: Joseph Rowntree.

Such a development of mutualism and cooperativeness also provides scope for community-led commissioning, by using CE techniques and a strategic programme of change management. This will encourage a joined up, user-led approach to health, housing and social care services and thus to integration of health, housing, education and social service delivery (Turning Point, 2011). It provides a form of values-based process, rooted in engaging sections of the community to develop 'connected care', essentially a way in which health, social care, education, housing and other key elements of local services can be constructed differently in an overlapping, intersecting, efficient and economical way.

5.7 Conclusion

Community engagement in all its forms is an essential prerequisite of effective focused commissioning of health and wellbeing. Participatory methods that engage and build capacity within communities and specific groups are therefore central to promoting mental wellbeing but only if they go beyond token involvement through dissemination of information to an active involvement in decision-making resulting in co-production. Only by engaging with communities is it possible realistically to understand what might improve wellbeing and how NHS and local authority resources can bring about improvements. This chapter has offered a number of ideas on CE, especially on the main objectives of any process, and on some of the pitfalls that may accompany CE programmes.

Notes

1 www.publicengagement.ac.uk/how/guides/community-engagement/resources (accessed 15 February 2013).

2 Involve, www.involve.org.uk, and for research see www.invo.org.uk (accessed 15 February 2013).

3 See, for example, a useful community engagement toolkit developed by Manchester City Council, www.manchester.gov.uk/site/scripts/download_info.php?downloadID=172 (accessed 15 February 2013).

4 Professor Celia Davies, LSE, Evidence to the Health Select Committee on Patient and Public Involvement, February 2007.

CHAPTER 6

Sweeping Shadows Away: Children, Adolescents and Future Adults

Without exception, current policy and the evidence point to the importance of intervening early with the benefits of doing so being realised across the life course. In this chapter we look at the importance of promoting the health and wellbeing of children by focusing on their parents.

6.1 Introduction

When we were researching the background to this book, everyone we spoke to said that preventing harms to children was the most important way to improve health and wellbeing for the children themselves as they grow and mature, for their peers and families and for wider society. From 'minus 9 months to 18 years' was the response of one third sector organisation's Chief Executive.[1] Prevention and health promotion for this group is possibly the most exciting and beneficial given that some 50% of adult mental health problems are considered to start before age 14, if not earlier.[2] Everyone wants to protect children from the worst aspects of parental misjudgements, to prevent sexual or physical abuse, to assist children to grow and develop, to prevent bullying and other adverse behaviours in school, and to enable children to mature into healthy and well-controlled adults. Paradoxically, placing an emphasis on children means giving a priority to working with adults. If we are to break through the cycle of disadvantage, challenge the prevailing attitudes towards parenting, develop child support and establish appropriate education, we will need an approach to the putative or actual parents of those children that changes their behaviours in order to change the lives of their children.

All the available evidence suggests that the health of mothers and fathers prenatally is vitally important. Maternal health before conception is important for a healthy baby; not smoking, or taking controlled drugs, or drinking during pregnancy are essential features of a healthy pregnancy and a healthy baby (Foresight, 2008). Recent research on prenatal depression suggests that it is a strong predictor of postnatal depression and has been associated with premature birth and low birth-weight, and with poor sleep patterns and less responsiveness in the baby. Children of mothers with depression or other mental health prenatal, perinatal and postnatal problems tend to have emotional and behavioural problems, which sometimes feeds through into adult problems (Field, 2011).

6.2 Early life chances: the effects of prenatal and postnatal depression and anxiety

There have been few antenatal interventions aimed at preparing women or men for the transition to parenthood. Earlier attempts to intervene antenatally to prevent postnatal depression and anxiety have had only limited impact. However, a recent study of a community network aiming to increase social support and access to health professionals (to facilitate treatment of existing antenatal depression or anxiety), demonstrated a successful outcome. By targeting risk factors for poor postnatal adjustment it was possible to achieve the dual aim of reducing both postnatal symptoms of depression or anxiety and parenting difficulties including a trend towards reduced parenting stress (Milgrom et al., 2011). Postnatal depression affects a mother's capability to care for her baby, restricts her ability to engage positively with the baby in social interactions (Murray and Cooper, 2003; Poobalan et al., 2007), and affects cognitive and emotional development of the child as it grows (Murray et al., 1996a, 1996b; Murray et al., 1999; Hay et al., 2003). Around 70,000 women experience postnatal depression to some degree in the UK each year (Glover and O'Connor, 2002) and studies of the early detection and treatment of postnatal depression have shown positive benefits for mothers (Appleby et al., 1997; Misri et al., 2000; Cooper et al., 2003).

The mental health of mothers is contingent upon an interaction between material, social, psychological and biological factors. Becoming a mother, and indeed a father, is a highly significant transition and a time of increased psychological vulnerability with the potential of childbirth to act as a major stressor (Riecher-Rosslier and Rhode, 2003, cited in Lewin, 2010). Unsurprisingly, many women experience postnatal blues, regarded as a normal variation of change occurring after childbirth (Miller and Ruckstalis, 1999 cited in Lewin, 2010). There are particular at-risk groups: teenagers where pregnancy might be associated with a complex background of sexual abuse and alcohol or substance abuse (Bayatpour et al., 1992), women who have experienced previous perinatal loss and women living in adverse social circumstances, particularly those exposed to domestic violence or using alcohol and illicit drugs, black Caribbean women living in the inner city (Edge, 2007) or those in prison.

However, there is evidence that the mother's postnatal depression has 'continuing negative effects on maternal interactions through childhood' (Murray et al., 2010: 1150), which contribute to poorer educational attainment at 16. After controlling for smoking, alcohol use, birth weight for gestational age, maternal age, sex of the child and socio-economic status, behavioural and emotional problems at age four were independently associated with antenatal anxiety in late pregnancy, not only with antenatal depression (O'Connor et al., 2002), although the odds ratios were only just significant. O'Connor et al.'s conclusion was that both antenatal anxiety and postnatal depression represent separate risks for behavioural and emotional problems in children. Similarly, Murray et al. (1999: 1259) found that although maternal behaviour varies according to circumstances, 'exposure to maternal depression in the early postpartum months may have an enduring influence on child psychological adjustment'. Kim-Cohen et al. (2003) identified from a study of 1116 twin pairs assessed at five and seven years of age that the combination of maternal depression and antisocial personality traits had the worst effect on antisocial behaviour in children. Kim-Cohen et al. (2003) observe that there are likely to be high levels of stress and disorganisation in these families, which may well be related to, and reflect, material hardship and reflect a lack of social and personal resources for managing in difficult contexts.

Accordingly, intervening to prevent or reduce prenatal and postnatal depression and the consequences for the children involved is likely to be cost-effective and lead to other outcomes, including improved educational and employment achievement and better parenting of subsequent generations. A systematic review of eight papers reporting clinical trials of methods to improve the mother–infant relationship demonstrated that, '[C]ognitive development in children of depressed mothers, along with better mother–infant relationships, might be improved with sustained interventions' (Poobalan et al., 2007: 378). Similarly, Tandon et al. (2011) found positive results of a cognitive behavioural intervention to prevent perinatal depression amongst home visiting clients, predominantly unmarried and unemployed African Americans. In a relatively small study, boys, but not girls, of mothers with postnatal depression obtained poorer educational results, as a result of effects on early child cognitive functioning, which showed strong continuity from infancy (Murray et al., 2010).

The above discussion does not imply that all the maternal problems are medical, far from it, with psychological difficulties reflecting a complex mix of childhood experiences, socioeconomic factors and quality of social support and relationships. However, the evidence for intervening early and addressing postnatal problems is relatively robust. In guidelines (2006, 2007a) NICE recommended that psychological therapy should be available for pregnant women who have symptoms of depression and/ or anxiety that do not meet diagnostic criteria but significantly interfere with personal and social functioning and who have had a previous episode of depression and/or anxiety. They further advised that managed clinical networks should be established for the delivery of perinatal mental health services that could bring an effective concentration of expertise, dedicated professional time, and explicit responsibility for the delivery of appropriate care to women with perinatal and postnatal depression (NICE, 2007a). Ammerman et al. (2010) suggest the need to include a measurement of depression into every home visit with a new mother (or a new mother-to-be), perhaps by a midwife in the perinatal period or a health visitor subsequently. Whilst this will generate savings in the long run, Ammerman et al. note that peer education (for example, on parenting skills) does not appear to work and that women need properly managed programmes offered by professional staff. Having said this, one of the problems of modern society is the breakdown of traditional social groups and the isolation of young mothers. In the past women learned from their mothers and from other women. Over-medicalising the needs of young parents is to be avoided and support for local women's groups is one way of encouraging health and wellbeing.

Breastfeeding is one maternal activity that is affected, either brought to a halt prematurely or stopped completely, by postnatal depression. Yet the benefits of breastfeeding are well known. Breastfeeding for less than six months (compared to greater than six months) is an independent predictor of mental health problems in childhood and adolescence (Oddy et al., 2010); and more recently it has been shown that breastfeeding for four months or more 'is associated with fewer behavioural problems in children at age 5' (Heikkilä et al., 2011: 635;

see also Gribble, 2006). Taken with the findings above, this points to the need to enhance the understanding and skills of midwives and health visitors in relation to the psychological health of women and their babies, and the role of other women in an area who have had children and can advise new mothers (for example, the charity Little Angels offers local breastfeeding support and has grown quickly in Lancashire and surroundings during the last five years, see www.littleangels.org.uk). Both professional staff and volunteers have a central role to play in supporting breastfeeding, identifying potential mental health problems, providing an appropriate level of social and psychological support, and signposting to effective professional help and being highly alert to the social context, taking action as appropriate.

Given the evidence about the importance of parenting skills training, it would seem appropriate to relate perinatal and postnatal care to early parenting skills development (Barlow and Coren, 2003). In other words a holistic approach is needed that recognises the woman's lifestyle and life-choices, her present accommodation, income, relationships (including other children) and possible employment demands, as well as her psychological or psychiatric condition. In a longitudinal study with 58 participants (and 42 controls), children of mothers with postnatal depression were found to be at increased risk themselves for depression by 16 years of age (Murray et al., 2011). This may be due to vulnerability within the child established in infancy and early childhood, by exposure to further maternal or family adversity. Murray et al. (2011) comment that routine screening for postnatal depression, and parenting support for mothers with postnatal depression, might reduce child and adolescent risk of clinical depression.

We must put down a marker at this point. Whilst prenatal, perinatal and postnatal care is very important and must continue to be strengthened and targeted, there is substantial evidence that a life course approach to health care is just as essential. During the 1970s, 1980s and 1990s, especially in the USA, there was an emphasis on prenatal care to the exclusion of the wider determinants of longer-term health and functioning (Pies et al., 2012). Using a life course model (e.g. Lu and Halfon, 2003) it can be seen that the differences in protective and risk factors between different groups of women (by age, ethnicity or socio-economic status) result in inequalities in birth outcomes, such as birth weight and infant mortality. A complex interplay exists between biological, behavioural, psychological, environmental, and social protective and risk factors that contribute to health outcomes (Pies et al., 2012: 650). This suggests a number of important strategies for all families, but especially for those subject to discrimination on grounds of ethnicity or socio-economic status. These include:

- improving health care, including preconception and prenatal care, for all whilst ensuring affirmative action in favour of women from lower socio-economic groups and from ethnic minorities where there is evidence of disproportionately poor care;
- assertively providing inter-conception care (between the end of one pregnancy and the start of another) for women with prior adverse pregnancy outcomes;
- expanding health care access over the life course for women from lower socio-economic groups and from ethnic minorities;
- strengthening families and communities of all women but especially those from lower socio-economic groups and from ethnic minorities, including the involvement of fathers in order to build reproductive social capital;
- enhancing systems coordination and integration for family support services and investing in community building and urban renewal;

- addressing social, educational and economic inequalities and providing support for working mothers and families, and to find routes out of poverty;
- tackling the racism inherent in poorer outcomes and ensuring that women from ethnic minorities are given all necessary resources (amended from Pies et al., 2012).

All these features should be the basis of a health and wellbeing strategy between CCGs and HWBs, taking a universal approach that demands both a universal programme that offers opportunities to all with appropriately targeted resources for those with greater needs. Tackling domestic abuse, for example, requires accessible information, heightened awareness amongst professional staff and women who have or may suffer abuse, and early identification of abuse or the threat of abuse.

6.3 Socio-economic factors in childhood

Children affected by major psychological stressors appear to suffer increased rates of morbidity and mortality from chronic diseases later in life. Studies of children raised in poverty (in the West) or those who suffer physical or sexual exploitation or mistreatment appear to embed stress biologically and have increased levels of vascular problems, auto-immune disorders and premature mortality (Miller et al., 2011a). Various theories have been developed to explain these dynamics, from biomedical (Miller et al., 2011a) via behavioural to social explanations (for example, Marmot, 2010). Behavioural problems include poor social relationships, mistrust of others, amplified fear of possible threats, poor self-control and unhealthy lifestyle choices. Nonetheless there is probably a connection between the inequalities theory (Wilkinson and Pickett, 2009) and the implication for children of families in lower socio-economic groups.

We can speculate that a holistic bio-psychosocial model may provide some of the answers (as presented assertively by Miller et al., 2011a), but whether stress gets under the skin, at a molecular level as asserted by Miller and colleagues is unclear (although the increased epigenetics revolution is slowly providing evidence that this may indeed occur – see, for example, Bell and Spector, 2011). Yet we know that black African-Caribbean young people raised in the inner city suffer a not dissimilar stress reaction and are much more vulnerable to mental illness and to experience adverse treatment by mental health services (for example see Tidyman et al., 2004; Sharpley et al., 2001; Greene et al., 2008). Families of low socio-economic status have limited material resources, poor living conditions, low job control and limited coping options (Evans, 2004; Evans and Kim, 2007), spend less time with their children, tend to have poorer parenting skills and may use discipline more punitively and less consistently (Leventhal and Brooks-Gunn, 2000).

Evidence is accumulating that socio-economic factors have as much if not more influence on health status than the equitable provision of health care (Hawkins et al., 2012). Data from the British National Child Development Study (which began in 1958) (Goodman et al., 2011) demonstrates that psychological and physical health problems in childhood have long-term effects on socio-economic status. Those with psychological problems in childhood were substantially affected in working and earning as adults and in intergenerational and within-generation social mobility. By the age of 50 adult family incomes were reduced by 28% with serious impacts on ability to work, marriage stability and the respondents' 'conscientiousness and agreeableness'.[3] Estimated effects of psychological problems were more substantial than physical health problems (Goodman et al., 2011: 6034) and included effects on memory, agreeableness, conscientiousness, emotional stability and reduced cognitive abilities. Whilst child maltreatment increases the risk of financial and employment related difficulties in adulthood (Zielinski, 2009), effective treatments that are 'targeted at lowering the risk of experiencing these psychological conditions ... are likely ... to be very cost effective' (Goodman et al., 2011: 6036).

Box 6.1   Case Example from Burnley (Lancashire Care NHS Foundation Trust)

'Right person, right place, right skills and at the right time'

The Chai Centre is a combined Children's Centre and Healthy Living Centre, located in the Daneshouse area of Burnley, within the top 2% deprivation in the country. The centre is a base for the Children's Centre Team, the Healthy Living Centre Team and the Children and Families Integrated Team (CFIT). Its core purpose is to improve the outcomes for young people and their families, with a particular focus on disadvantaged families, in order to reduce inequalities in child development and school readiness; to contribute to reducing health inequalities, promoting healthy eating and wellbeing messages by offering diet and nutrition advice; and the CFIT 0–19 service delivers all aspects of the Health Child programme in the locality. The universal and holistic nature of the service ensures that all community staff can interact readily and appropriately.

- Children's Centre services are delivered mainly through universal visits to all families with a child under five, group sessions at the centre and in local schools and community settings geared to achieving the five every child matters outcomes (stay safe, be healthy, enjoy and achieve, positive contribution, achieve economic wellbeing).

- The Healthy Living Centre provides opportunities for affordable and culturally sensitive physical activity (gym, exercise classes, walks), promoting healthy eating (café, cook and eat groups, breastfeeding and weaning support), working in partnership with other departments and organisations to provide further health promotion opportunities, e.g. smoking cessation, sexual health and mental wellbeing, and to signpost centre users into other services provided elsewhere as appropriate.

- The CFIT is integrated with Action on Children's Accident Project, Paediatric Liaison and clerical support to provide an integrated and holistic approach working alongside the Immunisation and Vaccination Team. The service provides both universal and targeted interventions.

- The Healthy Living service is provided mainly within the centre, and has robust links with schools, the school nurses delivering the healthy child programme 5–19, National Child Measuring Programme, vaccinations, targeted interventions and health needs assessments in all schools. An enhanced version of the Healthy Child Programme has been developed with every family receiving 12 core home visits in the first three years of life. These are boosted by bespoke packages of care jointly delivered to families with assessed additional needs. Health visitors and Children's Centre workers undertake some joint visits, particularly with more complex issues. Where Children's Centre workers provide family support, the health visitor is always fully informed and provides continuing guidance.

The centre's integrated approach has ensured that:

- safeguarding issues are less likely to be missed and problems are spotted sooner;

- health visitors have assisted Children's Centre staff develop their skills and the Children's Centre team has helped health visitors by delivering continuing support to more deprived families, working effectively in an ethnically diverse area;

- the intensive outreach programme led to a dramatic increase in families accessing services at the centre and very high levels of engagement are maintained;

- integrated working has allowed the teams to use the mix of skills effectively – families are supported by the worker with the right skills and knowledge for them, freeing health visitors to concentrate on the most complex issues.

Research on the social determinants of health has rapidly become an all-embracing business as the results of the WHO Commission and the Marmot Review (2010) in the UK have drawn attention to the relevance of socio-economic factors in the aetiology of disease; and the ability of individuals and communities to deal with the implications of disease is also affected by social factors. In a recent publication, EuroHealthNet has identified the implications of what it terms the 'gradient in health' (Stegeman and Costongs, 2012: 5). People with a lower educational attainment, poorer income or less attractive occupations tend to die at a lower age. Research suggests it is very difficult to reverse the effects of early disadvantage and thus it is better to improve the health and wellbeing of all children as early as possible, especially focusing on those from the lowest socio-economic groups. Even after adjusting for socio-economic status, childhood poverty in all its forms is a good predictor of adult health. Life expectancy at birth and age 65 varies considerably by social class, as shown in Figures 6.1 and 6.2.

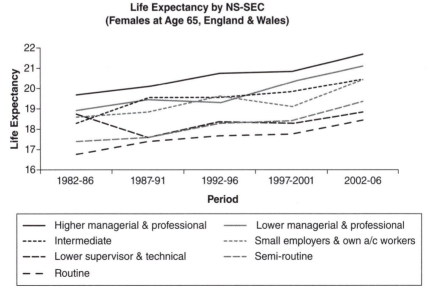

Figure 6.1 Life expectancy of females at age 65, by social class in England and Wales

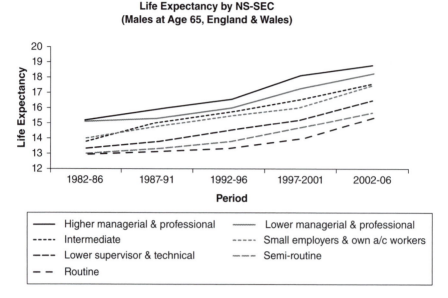

Figure 6.2   Life expectancy of males at age 65, by social class in England and Wales

Environment is a significant influence on early childhood development. Cumulative exposure to physical, intellectual, social, familial and emotional distress all take their toll. Children's wellbeing depends mainly on the 'quality of their family environment' (Stegeman and Costongs, 2012: 31). Indeed four major factors jointly and severally affect life chances and opportunities: family income, family structure, parental support and skill, and cultural capital (Esping-Andersen, 2007). Consequently providing support to families in the early years has a much larger payback than might be envisaged. By investing time and energy into those poorer families with babies and infants we will be able to ensure that we break the 'cycle of disadvantage' so graphically described by Sir Keith Joseph in 1972[4] (Welshman, 2007).

Income and wealth disparities have a significant effect on health; the health of children and adolescents is no exception. For example, Figure 6.3 shows subjective health status measured against 'wealth'. The graph for Sweden is less steep than for the UK or Slovenia, suggesting that the disparities of income and wealth are less severe in Sweden, even though subjective health is highest for the most well off in the UK. This fits with what we would expect of the social democratic and egalitarian aspects of those societies (taken from Stegeman and Costongs, 2012). Pioneering work by Wilkinson and Pickett (2009) has demonstrated convincingly that income or poverty gradients are intimately associated with a number of important health outcomes. They demonstrate the impact on child wellbeing of their estimate of the income equality gradient. Why the UK has such low child wellbeing deserves some discussion.

Wilkinson and Pickett used a dimension of *subjective* wellbeing measured by the following indicators in the UNICEF child wellbeing scale:

- Health
  - ○ Young people rating their own health only 'fair' or 'poor'
- School life
  - ○ Young people 'liking school a lot'

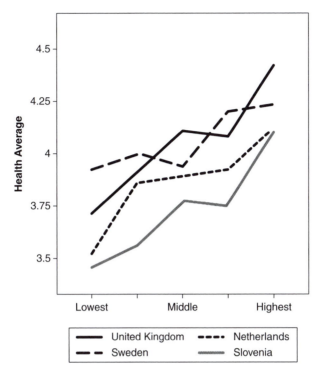

Figure 6.3   Disparities of income lead to wider gaps between rich and poor on subjective health

- Personal wellbeing
   - Children rating themselves above the mid-point of a 'Life Satisfaction Scale'
- Children reporting negatively about personal wellbeing

From the Innocenti Report Card No. 7 (UNICEF, 2007) we can see that the UK is doing very badly in comparison to all Western countries on the six dimensions of wellbeing used. The *material* child wellbeing measure includes relative income poverty, absolute income poverty, households without jobs, reported deprivation, few educational resources, fewer than ten books at home and low family affluence (although a note of caution should be included as the use of indicators may be limited by data availability and quality). Using this particular dimension is important because, as we saw above, there is evidence from many countries that children who experience childhood poverty are, on average, more vulnerable. They are, generally, more likely to be in poor health, to have learning and behavioural difficulties, to underachieve in school, to become pregnant at an early age, to have lower skills and aspirations, to be low paid, unemployed and welfare dependent.[5] Health outcomes are affected by socio-economic characteristics of parents and are superior for children of parents with higher socio-economic status. Of the six wellbeing dimensions (material wellbeing, health and safety, educational wellbeing, family and peer relationships, behaviours and risks, and subjective wellbeing) the UK scores moderately on only one, and does badly on the other five. This begs the question: is inequality the main driver of these poor scores or are there other factors involved (Welshman, 2007)?

Table 6.1   Child wellbeing and inequality

Country	Child wellbeing ranking from the UNICEF index	Inequality rating. Higher score = greater equality
Netherlands	4.2	8
Sweden	5	7
Denmark	7.2	8
Finland	7.5	8
Spain	8	5
Switzerland	8.3	8
Norway	8.7	7
Italy	10	3
Ireland	10.2	7
Belgium	10.7	5
Germany	11.2	6
Canada	11.8	6
Greece	11.8	3
Poland	12.3	6
Czech Republic	12.5	5
France	13	6
Portugal	13.7	6
Austria	13.8	6
Hungary	14.5	5
United States	18	3

Source: UNICEF (2007) *Child Poverty in Perspective: An Overview of Child Well-being in Rich Countries. A Comprehensive Assessment of the Lives and Well-being of Children and Adolescents in the Economically Advanced Nations*, Innocenti Report Card No. 7. UNICEF, Innocenti Research Centre, Florence, available at: http://www.unicef-irc.org/publications/pdf/rc7_eng.pdf and UNICEF (2010) *The Children Left Behind: A League Table of Inequality in Child Well-being in the World's Rich Countries*, Innocenti Report Card No. 9. UNICEF, Innocenti Research Centre, Florence, available at: http://www.unicef-irc.org/publications/pdf/rc9_eng.pdf.

6.4 Sexual and physical abuse in childhood

Sexual and physical abuse in childhood is also related to poorer mental health and wellbeing in adults. Sexual abuse has been found to be consistently associated with increases in risks of later mental health problems, whilst exposure to physical abuse showed weaker and less consistent effects (Fergusson et al., 2008). These findings suggest that much of the association between childhood physical abuse and later mental health 'reflects the general family context in which childhood physical abuse occurs' (Fergusson et al., 2008: 607). In an earlier paper, the same researchers found 'pervasive bivariate associations between exposure to childhood sexual abuse and physical abuse and a range of educational outcomes spanning high school and university achievement. For all outcomes there were clear and linear trends for increasing severity of both [forms of abuse] exposure to be associated with decreasing educational achievement' (Boden et al., 2007: 1111). However, the authors note that a number of covariate factors confounded the results suggesting that poorer educational attainment reflected the psychosocial context within which the abuse occurred; nor did they find gender effects which had been seen elsewhere (for example, see Myerson et al., 2002; Thompson et al., 2004).

We need to link these findings with the discussion of intimate partner violence. Taylor et al. (2009) reported that, in a study of intimate partner violence and maternal risk factors with the risk of maternal child maltreatment, mothers reported 'an average of 25 acts of psychological aggression and 17 acts of physical aggression against their 3-year-old children in the year before the study, 11% reported some act of neglect toward their children during the same period'. Intimate partner violence and maternal parenting stress were both consistent risk factors for psychological aggression, physical aggression, spanking and neglect. Sexual and physical abuse in childhood is associated with poorer educational attainment often reflecting a neglectful and abusing environment rather than the abuse per se.

6.5 Domestic abuse and intimate partner violence

Although we are primarily concerned with health and wellbeing from a positive perspective, depression and severe anxiety, as well as more serious injuries and physical disorders, undermine any conception of wellbeing for some women who are abused by their partners.

Preliminary evidence from a number of studies suggests that frequent exposure to domestic abuse is an independent risk factor for depressive symptoms amongst late adolescents and young adults (Cross et al., 2012). Results support a renewed call for (a) increased attention to depression amongst children exposed to adults' interpersonal violence, and (b) greater efforts to bridge prevention and intervention efforts regarding domestic violence and child maltreatment (Russell et al., 2010). One study in Brazil evaluated whether the probability of postpartum depression (PPD) increases with an upward gradient of intimate partner violence (IPV) during pregnancy and whether substance use by either member of the couple modified this relationship. What the research found was that there was no increase in depression beyond the first violent episode when neither party had abused alcohol, but once partners' alcohol abuse was included the levels of depression steadily increased as the violence continued from the second episode onwards (Lobato et al., 2012; but see also Forrester and Harwin, 2010). Both these studies suggest there should be tailored preventive, screening and intervention procedures for IPV and alcohol misuse during pregnancy and the postpartum period, which is then followed, if necessary, into adolescence (Lobato et al., 2012). Furthermore, good practice points to the importance of not only focusing on the mother but also listening to other children and providing effective support to the, usually male, perpetrator (see a range of publications at the National Academy of Parenting Practitioners;[6] Hunter, 2011).

Exposure to violence and traumatic events during childhood has long been associated with poor physical and psychological health during adulthood. For example, Kuhlman et al. (2012) found that children exposed to IPV with post-traumatic stress indications had fewer overall health problems but did have asthma and gastrointestinal problems that were considered to be symptoms of poor psychological adjustment using mother-reported symptoms. It also appears that exposure to IPV is under reported. Mandatory reporting can increase the number of cases that come to the attention of child welfare agencies, but without resources for training and programming may do more harm than good as it can lead to inappropriate reporting, lack of referral for further assessment and strains on the child welfare system (Taft et al., 2009).

As we have seen briefly, empirical data are limited, but current research and practice suggest that child welfare agencies seeking to improve ways of tackling exposure to IPV need to collaborate with other disciplines involved with preventing and responding to IPV, mobilise the necessary resources to support training and programming, consider methods that avoid stigmatising parents, and build in a programme evaluation component to increase knowledge about effective practice. This crosses the boundaries of health and social care, engages GPs and the primary health care team and local authority safeguarding teams. It is a prime candidate on which CCGs and HWBs should concentrate and identify how to mainstream evidence-based interventions as well as reorienting the practice of the existing workforce to focus on parental mental health.

6.6 Parenting skills

Various strategies have been developed to improve child health and longer-term functioning. One of those is to emphasisie programmes that support parents and children adequately, such as Sure Start (Belsky et al., 2006). Another is to improve parenting for all with specific targeted approaches to those identified as at risk. As we have seen, children raised in poverty do less well than children raised in more favourable circumstances on a range of measures of attainment and quality of life (Scott et al., 2006). Providing access to parenting skills classes for everyone ensures that those who may think they don't need help have as much chance as anyone else to obtain support and ideas to improve their knowledge. But for parents living in relative deprivation, and/or where the woman has postnatal depression, and/or a learning disability or other disabling condition, there is an opportunity to 'drill down' and offer targeted facilities geared to their local and specific circumstances. 'Suboptimal' parenting is a risk factor for a wide range of health, social and educational outcomes (see, for example, Petrie et al., 2007), but many parenting programmes in the past have been based largely on behaviour management strategies (Bonin et al., 2011).

To address the overtly behavioural nature of parenting support in the 1990s and earlier, the last decade has seen those programmes supplemented with a focus on family relationships, such as the Family Links Nurturing Programme developed in the UK (Simkiss et al., 2010), the Strengthening Families, Strengthening Communities programme (Wilding and Barton, 2007, 2009; Lindsay et al., 2008), the Incredible Years programme (Webster-Stratton, 2006; 2007; Webster-Stratton and Reid, 2009), and the Triple P – Positive Parenting Program (Sanders, 1999). The Strengthening Families Strengthening Communities (SFSC) programme was developed in the USA, predominantly to enhance the development of effective parenting skills in minority ethnic groups. The course includes cultural and spiritual dimensions, enhancing relationships, rites of passage and community involvement (Lindsay et al., 2008).

The Incredible Years is a USA programme for groups of parents of children aged 0–8 years, and focuses on enhancing effective, positive parenting, in order to enable children's development and education and to manage behavioural problems where necessary (Webster-Stratton, 2007). In addition the programme emphasises parents' adaptation so they are more able to manage their own problems and relationships. There is substantial evidence that the programme works (see, for example, Gardner et al., 2006). The Triple P – Positive Parenting Program was developed in Australia. It differs from other parenting programmes in comprising a complex system of interventions grouped into five levels, reflecting increasing complexity and severity of need. It enables parents to provide a safe and interesting environment for their children, a positive learning environment and assertive discipline, while maintaining realistic expectations and taking care of themselves as parents (Lindsay et al., 2008).

In the study by Lindsay and colleagues, all three programmes achieved significant improvements on all measures with effect sizes ranging from 0.57 to 0.93 for parenting style; from 0.33 to 0.77 for parenting satisfaction and self-efficacy; and from 0.49 to 0.88 for parental mental wellbeing. However, the Strengthening Families Strengthening Communities was 'significantly less effective than both the other two programmes in improving parental efficacy, satisfaction and mental wellbeing'. The study sample was predominantly white and did not reflect the ethnic mix in society, and this may have been relevant to the way the programme was received. There were also significant improvements in child behaviour as a result of all the programmes, with effect sizes for reduction in conduct problems from –0.44 to –0.71 (Lindsay et al., 2008).

Founded on social learning theory, the Incredible Years programme consists of at least 12 weekly, two-hour group sessions delivered by skilled practitioners. Using a collaborative approach (that includes role play, group discussion, homework and reviewing DVDs of family behaviour) the programme encouraged parents to learn from each other, in order to:

- promote positive parenting;
- improve parent–child relationships;
- reduce critical and physical discipline and increase the use of positive strategies;
- help parents to identify social learning theory principles for managing behaviour;
- improve home–school relationships. (McDaniel et al., 2010: 2)

Parenting affects social competences and educational achievement, as well as employment opportunities and thus income in later life. A study undertaken by the Institute of Psychiatry and published by the Joseph Rowntree Foundation demonstrated some valuable improvements to the Incredible Years programme by combining it with a reading pro-gramme (Primary Age Learning Study (PALS), Scott et al., 2006). Describing an evaluation of the factors influencing the effectiveness of a parenting intervention in one of the poorest parts of Britain, the authors conceded that ensuring a child is raised 'experiencing warmth, love and encouragement within safe boundaries is far harder for parents who live in the stressful conditions found in poor neighbourhoods' (Scott et al., 2006: 1, see also Scott et al., 2010). The intervention improved several aspects of parenting in important ways, such as increasing sensitive responding to children, improving the use of appropriate discipline and decreasing criticism. Proportionate universalism[7] enables implementation that offers uni-versal interventions alongside targeted mechanisms. As the authors conclude, most fami-lies, even in highly disadvantaged areas, live without problems in cohesive communities. Targeting interventions by geography, ethnicity or socio-economic group may waste money. To maximise effectiveness, it is essential to assess direct indicators of need for inter-ventions. Similarly a study by Edwards et al. (2007) suggested that the Incredible Years parenting programme would be most cost-effective for children at the highest risk of devel-oping conduct disorders (see also Barrett, 2010).

Although a lot of what we say here is concerned with positive approaches to parenting skills it is worth noting the rather negative psychiatric evaluation of poor parenting. A systematic narrative analysis of 23 papers on 16 cohorts of children and parents, published between 1970 and 2008, found that abusive relationships predicted depression, anxiety and post-traumatic stress disorder, and maternal emotional unavailability in early life predicted suicide attempts in adolescence. Given the importance of common psychiatric problems, these studies highlighted the need to minimise harm associated with dysfunctional parent–child relationships (Weich et al., 2011). On the other hand, if children are brought up with warm, firm, encouraging parenting, the evidence is clear that they can succeed even in more adverse circumstances (Scott et al., 2006).

Child poverty is a key determinant of poor educational achievement largely due to the effects of economic deprivation on the mental and emotional health of adolescents. Adolescent emotional wellbeing is a strong predictor of educational achievement and emotional wellbeing, and 'mediates the relationship between poverty and educational achievement' (Sznitman et al., 2011). Ameliorating the adverse effects of early deprivation is likely to have an impact both on educational achievement and subjective wellbeing (Sznitman et al., 2011). Whilst good childcare cannot alone deal with the effects of deprivation or childhood poverty, improvements in social capital can be achieved from a combination of childcare centres and improved community coalition building. Children appear to do better than expected because their mothers are benefitting directly from superior access to assets and social networks that are promoted both by the childcare centres themselves and the local partnerships that connect the centres. In resilient communities, 'a more functional coalition increases the production of social capital that is typical of childcare centres, leading to greater maternal wellbeing, which in turn leads to better children's mental health' (Maggi et al., 2011: 1087).

A debate continues over the cost-effectiveness of additional health visitor interventions delivered to women postnatally. One study in which health visitors delivered psychological therapies to women at high risk of postnatal depression showed a 90% chance that the cost per quality adjusted life year (QALY) gained would be less than £30,000 (considered the threshold for cost-effectiveness by NICE) (Morrell et al., 2009, quoted in McDaid and Park, 2011). However, earlier studies have shown little benefit, such as the studies by Wiggins et al. (2005a; 2005b) of supportive home visits to ethnically diverse mothers in London. These studies to some degree bear out Olds's (2002) contention that home visiting by 'paraprofessionals' is not as effective as that by clinically informed staff. One meta-analysis reported that generally home visiting programmes lead to improvements in the quality of the home environment, but unfortunately few of the studies reported were from the UK (Kendrick et al., 2000). Conversely the work of voluntary/third sector organisations locally often demonstrates valuable improvements and is well liked by service users.

6.7 Adolescent health: self-esteem and bullying

We have seen that early childhood experiences have significant effects on later development. Early deprivation leads to mental and emotional problems, poorer educational attainment, to bullying or being bullied at school, and to tobacco, alcohol and drug abuse. Intervening as early as possible to ameliorate the effects of income and emotional poverty in childhood can lead to substantial improvements in health and also save significant amounts of money (see Chapter 9 on cost-effectiveness of interventions). Schools are one of the most important institutions in which to tackle emotional health of adolescents – promoting self-esteem and preventing bullying. An early example was demonstrated by the Mind 'Myself' project that sought to assist teachers in five Newcastle schools to work with their pupils in an innovative, pastoral and supportive way (Stewart and Brownlow, 1985).

Similar schemes are likely to be valued by pupils and students and should be introduced as part of a whole school's commitment to supporting students' emotional health, helping those in distress and improving the physical and psychosocial environment. Unfortunately, emotional health does not appear to be given sufficient time within the curriculum, and although support is available to students in distress the quality and quantity varies markedly, especially in a school's response to bullying (Kidger et al., 2009). Put in technical language, school bullying in both primary and secondary schools has an adverse effect on personal 'capital accumulation', in school and later. The adverse effects of bullying appear to be greater if it occurs nearer to examination times; and bullying affects both the perpetrator and the victim. Educational attainment is poorer for the perpetrator but the effects on lifetime earnings are more persistent for those subject to bullying (Brown and Taylor, 2008).

In a paper for NICE, Hummel et al. (2009) undertook a review of 40 papers that met their inclusion criteria, notably (a) randomised control trials (RCTs) or other robust study designs, (b) impact and (c) applicability to the UK. The majority of papers (30) addressed bullying and disruptive behaviours and a rather smaller number focused on promotion of positive social behaviour. Bullying is now spreading to new technology, with on-line bullying through Facebook, Twitter and other websites, and demands attention from parents as well as further research on its effects and mechanisms to curb these harmful behaviours. Overall, the review offered mixed conclusions. Many of the papers were of research conducted in the USA or other countries with relatively few from the UK; and a sizeable proportion of the USA papers were of schools with large numbers of African Americans, which the authors considered to be less replicable in the UK (Hummel et al., 2009: 11). Although there was meagre evidence that the interventions achieved lasting positive social behaviours (i.e. beyond one year at grade 8 or 9), nonetheless conflict resolution training promoted improved social competence in the short term (Stevahn, 2002) and programmes involving peer mediators were successful over a longer period. Evidence on preventing bullying was more mixed with differing emphases on the roles of peers, teachers, external agencies, community and parents. One programme that was successful was a computer-based anti-bullying curriculum that led to a fourfold drop in those saying they would engage in bullying behaviour (Evers et al., 2007). Whether this was likely to be sustained was unclear.

Personality seems to shape much of the students' responses to bullying as well as their emotional health and wellbeing. Danilo Garcia, in a study of 289 secondary school students in Sweden, found that three of the 'Big Five' personality traits were strongly related to wellbeing, and that self-directedness was strongly correlated with subjective wellbeing and life satisfaction (Garcia, 2011).[8] Interventions to improve students' self-directedness and self-confidence could have significant paybacks; by self-directedness we mean the ability to regulate and adapt behaviour to the demands of a situation, to be confident, reliable, responsible, resourceful and goal-oriented. Programmes that encourage these traits in students will both attenuate bullying behaviours and give students the resources to stand up to those who would become bullies. Many of those who are bullied either start with low self-esteem or it is forced upon them by their experiences (Liu et al., 2004). Low self-esteem is associated with many mental health problems that often become a vicious circle – the more depressed or anxious a person becomes the more their opinion of themselves reduces and the more they avoid experiences that might help rebuild their self-esteem. Most of the research on low self-esteem has suggested that the most promising treatment outcomes have been with cognitive behavioural therapy (CBT) (a process that helps individuals identify ways in which a person interacts with the way they feel and what they can do about it) (Fennell, 2009). Poor parenting can lead to low self-esteeem in older adolescents and young adults if not obviated early, which is why we have spent some time considering early childhood and parenting experiences. Many conditions later in life can be traced back to low self-esteem, poor self-management, and reduced concern with personal care. As we shall see in Chapter 8, diabetes is a classic example of the way low self-esteem generates a poor quality of life that leads either to depression or diabetes (or both) but which is causative is unclear.

6.8 Healthy or health promoting schools

One valuable way to improve the way in which schools provide support to pupils is to focus on health knowledge and improvements in healthy lifestyles. The health promoting school (HPS), ideas for which have been in operation since the late 1990s, is one that continually 'strengthens its capacity as a healthy setting for living, learning and working' (WHO Global School Health Initiative, 2005).[9] The HPS is a school that fosters health and learning, engages the whole educational community in efforts to make the school a healthy place, strives to provide a healthy environment, and implements policies and practices that respect an individual's wellbeing and dignity. Healthy schools work to improve the health of those in the school, and work with community leaders to help them understand how the community contributes to, or undermines, health and education. Health promoting schools focus on caring for oneself and others, making healthy decisions and taking control over one's life circumstances, creating conditions conducive to health, building capacity for social justice, and working with health and social care to encourage health promotion and prevention initiatives.

In Australia the HPS has been an objective for some time as a way of influencing health-related behaviours. In 1995 the World Health Organization defined a health promoting school as one in which:

> all members of the school community work together to provide pupils with integrated and positive experiences and structures, which promote and protect their health. This includes both the formal and the informal curriculum in health, the creation of a safe and healthy school environment, the provision of appropriate health services and the involvement of the family and wider community in efforts to promote health.

The healthy schools framework is built on three inter-related areas (see Figure 6.4): teaching and learning curriculum, school environment, and partnerships and community links. Research to date on the efficacy and value of HPSs has shown mixed cost-effectiveness evidence as a result of the paucity of primary research, although the concept seems entirely right. The approach has been successful in improving some aspects of health – nutritional intake and fitness – and there was some evidence that the healthy schools initiative has impacted positively on aspects of mental and social wellbeing, particularly self-esteem and bullying, which have previously proved difficult to influence (Lister-Sharp et al., 1999). Systematic reviews of effectiveness were available for nutrition and exercise, safety, psychological aspects of health, sexual health, substance use and personal hygiene. Almost all the interventions covered in the *Health Technology Assessment* review (Lister-Sharp et al., 1999) demonstrated improved health knowledge, but the impact of interventions on attitudes, health-related behaviour and health was much less reliable.

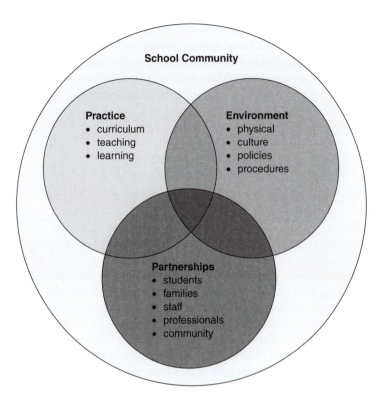

Figure 6.4 Health Promoting School image from the Australian Women and Children's Health Network, Centre for Health Promotion. Reproduced by kind permission of the Centre for Health Promotion

---

Box 6.2   Strengthening Families: case example from York

Holgate School in York used the Strengthening Families initiative to tackle alcohol usage. It adopted a 'whole school approach' – one that addressed simultaneously leadership, management and managing change, policy development, learning and teaching, curriculum planning and resourcing, school culture and environment, and giving children and young people a voice. By developing wellbeing partnerships with parents/carers and local communities, and assessing, recording and reporting the achievement of children and young people in a positive way they were able not only to reduce alcohol consumption but also to improve the overall wellbeing of the pupils. The programme is a seven-week family skills training programme designed to increase resilience and reduce risk factors for alcohol and substance misuse. After separate sessions for parents/carers and young people, they then work together and learn how to negotiate boundaries and reach practical agreements. Reviews of alcohol prevention interventions for young people have singled this programme out as one of the very few that has been proved to create long-term behavioural change in terms of reduced alcohol consumption. Research has also shown that the programme reduces aggressive and hostile behaviour, improves parent–child interaction and increases school attendance and attainment. (See at www.mystrongfamily.org.)

One important aspect of healthy schools is achieving reductions in alcohol consumption. NICE found evidence that two programmes (Strengthening Families, and Botvin's Life Skills Training) can produce long-term reductions in alcohol consumption; and two classroom-based programmes that targeted 12 and 13 year olds achieved medium- to long-term reductions in drinking and drink related behaviours, although a health educator-led programme appeared to be less successful (Jones et al., 2007). There are also opportunities to address the wider determinants of poor mental health at an individual level, for example future indebtedness, through developing the financial literacy of children and young people.

Of course, other interventions will be needed alongside these to tackle wholesale the problems of alcohol (see Chapter 7) and financial exclusion (see Leeds City Council).[10]

Box 6.3   Financial literacy: case example from Leeds

As part of its financial inclusion strategy, Leeds City Council has developed programmes on financial capability. These include work with young children, as well as programmes for primary schools and older children. It is relatively easy to work with children and young people of school age and more difficult to reach the adults most in need of help to understand their finances. The partners in the project had explicit health improvement goals and developed a number of initiatives targeted at children and young people including a range of enterprise programmes for young people from 10 to 14 and from 14 to 16 years. The aim is to develop financial skills in a real-life context. They impart a real understanding of how business works through helping young people to run their own or a simulated business. The Social Enterprise programme runs throughout the year. It enables children from age 6 to 16 to run their own social enterprise, benefiting their community. Young people make all decisions relating to the running of the business, including all financial accounting.

6.9 Conclusion

From a life course perspective, what happens to infants and children in their early years has implications for their whole lives (Halfon et al., 2005). Many of the problems we discuss in this book have a root in early upbringing. It is therefore unsurprising that not only do we emphasise early years interventions, but that they are also highly cost-effective. The problems of poor parenting can be alleviated, as can pre- and postnatal depression in mothers, and the distress and suffering associated with domestic (or intimate partner) violence, physical and sexual abuse of children, or parents being regularly drunk at home cause continuing complications for decades to come if not resolved. Adolescent bullying, poor educational attainment, difficulties in finding a job, poor self-management both leading to and continuing with a variety of disorders, and indeed the likely onset of major diseases such as stroke or CHD, all have their beginnings in early childhood distress. This chapter has covered some but by no means all the ground. It is the one area (despite our focus in later chapters on other matters) that we emphasise most strongly and to which we believe all commissioners should give careful attention.

Notes

1 Dr Andrew McCulloch, Chief Executive of the Mental Health Foundation speaking to Chris Heginbotham in 2009.

2 NAMI: The US National Alliance on Mental Illness, at www.nami.org/Template.cfm?Section= About_Mental_Illnes (accessed 29 June 2013).

3 Respondents were seen at birth and at ages 7, 11, 16, 23, 33, 42, 46 and 50. Psychological health (emotional maladjustment) was captured at 7 and 16, and parents' reports captured whether the child had been seen by a psychologist or psychiatrist at 11 and 16. Emotional maladjustment was rated on a five point scale and only moderate or severe maladjustment was counted (Goodman et al., 2011).

4 Sir Keith Joseph was a member of the Conservative Party Cabinet 1970–74. In 1972 he made a famous 'cycle of disadvantage' speech, examining his own family background, his concern with 'problem families' and the wider policy context of the early 1970s.

5 See www.unicef-irc.org/publications/pdf/rc7_eng.pdf (accessed 23 March 2013).

6 www.parentingresearch.org.uk/Publications.aspx (accessed 18 January 2013).

7 The term proportionate universalism was 'coined to highlight the assertion that in order to reduce the steepness of the social gradient within health, actions taken must be universal but with a scale and intensity that is proportionate to the level of disadvantage' (Marmot, 2010: 15).

8 The Big Five factors of personality are broad domains or dimensions that are used to describe human personality; the theory based on the Big Five factors is called the Five Factor Model (FFM) (Costa and McCrae, 1990; 1992). The Big Five framework of personality traits has emerged as a robust model for understanding the relationship between personality and various behaviours. The factors are: openness (inventive/curious vs. consistent/cautious); conscientiousness (efficient/organised vs. easy-going/careless); extraversion (outgoing/energetic vs. solitary/reserved); agreeableness (friendly/compassionate vs. cold/unkind); neuroticism (sensitive/nervous vs. secure/confident).

9 At www.who.int/school_youth_health/gshi/en/ (accessed 17 December 2012).

10 www.leeds.gov.uk/residents/Pages/Financial-Inclusion-Project.aspx (accessed 15 February 2013).

CHAPTER 7

Adults, Employment and Alcohol

This chapter covers work, worklessness and health and considers the use and abuse of alcohol as one of the critical features of adult wellbeing that affects work and also impinges on many people's lives.

7.1 Introduction

We have seen that early childhood trauma, poor parenting and social problems such as homelessness all contribute to a cycle of deprivation with long-term consequences. Distressed children grow into distressed or at least usually less competent adults. Whilst it is not true that if you are born poor you remain poor all your life – indeed there are many examples in which the stimulus of a financially poor but (possibly) psychologically rewarding family life leads to aggressively taken opportunities later – nonetheless there is good evidence that economically poorer families have problems later as adults in securing and retaining jobs and the wider benefits of society. It remains true that good early experiences, resources and opportunities offer tangible results in school performance, university attendance and employment opportunities. The present government's continued attacks on the poorest in society whilst rewarding the richest with tax reductions is at best unhealthy and at worst demonstrates a complete lack of understanding of the pressure and possibilities in today's society. As Wilkinson and Pickett (2009) have shown, increasing economic inequality is directly correlated with increased social inequality and a host of other social problems.

This chapter considers workplace mental and physical health, the benefits and opportunities to be obtained from focusing on workplace arrangements, and some of the problems and solutions of disorders that often (though not invariably) start at work.

Many workers when asked applauded an organisation's owners' or managers' interest in health and wellbeing at work, but a substantial number (around 30% depending on the study considered) resented the managers' or owners' interference in anything that was not directly concerned with workplace occupational health (DH, 2009c). This is understandable but is nonetheless unhelpful. Being able to address staff at work means we have a 'captive' audience with whom various lifestyle or wellbeing interventions can be

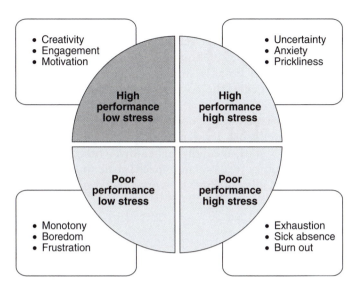

Figure 7.1   Performance–stress relationships (the target is to be as high as possible in the darker quadrant)

discussed; but it must be done ethically and responsibly, taking account of any objections raised by staff and recognising the specific circumstances and managerial relationships within a firm.

To some degree this goes to the heart of our concept of health, possibly more important in this section than elsewhere. As we saw in Chapter 2, health is one of those words, a bit like 'time', that we use frequently and think we understand, but which we find very difficult to define or explain. As the Hastings Center Report (Mordacci and Sobel, 1998: 34) described it, '[P]hysiological measurements alone fail to capture the subjective dimension of health. "Health" is an end *and* a means – it is a foundation for achievement, a first achievement itself, and a precondition for further achievement'.

'Health' is thus three things in one: the basis for a decent life, an objective itself and the necessary prerequisite for additional accomplishments. Health is also a broad term that encompasses social, psychological, environmental, political and economic factors. If we narrow it too much we will miss much that is relevant. By considering 'health' from a managerial or corporate perspective we may understate the important properties of 'health' that business does not wish to notice. Only a fully comprehensive and inclusive definition will capture the essence of why health matters in the workplace, and why employment should be more than simply a way to earn a living, important as that is.

Health and wellbeing in the workplace have improved enormously over the last 50 years. Fatal accidents have reduced by 50% (see Figure 7.2) in the last 20 years, but around 2.1 million people suffer work-related stress, and this has stayed more or less stable over the last ten years (see Figure 7.3). The recent implications of macro-economic policy are difficult to gauge. Will it lead to more stress at work for those concerned that they may lose their jobs; or will the overall reductions in employment lead to reductions in stress at work, only to see an increase in those unemployed with stress?

In 2001–2002, the cost to society of illness and injury at work was between £20 billion and £30 billion per annum – a huge sum of money that would repay preventive and health promoting activity (HSE, 2004 quoted from DH , 2009c). We can assume the amounts will have remained broadly similar ten years on. Although there has been a reduction in fatal accidents, the cost of dealing with workplace stress has continued to rise.

We are concerned in this chapter with good employment practices as well as with interventions to improve wellbeing in the workforce. Poor HR policy, lack of appropriate pastoral care for staff, mentally unhealthy working arrangements, low salaries and minimum statutory wages, and mechanistic programmes with little opportunity for advancement, all contribute to work-related stress, which in turn can

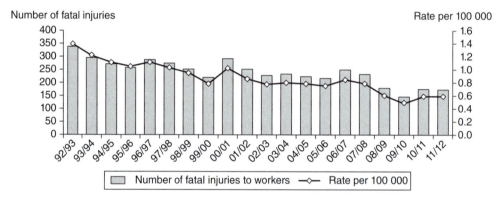

Figure 7.2 Number and rate of fatal injury to workers, 1992/93–2011/12

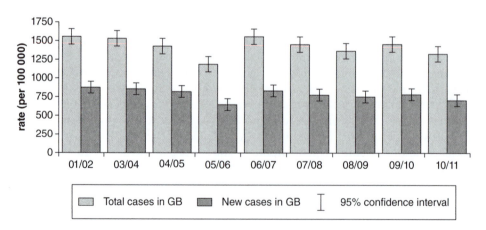

Figure 7.3 Total number of cases (prevalence) of workplace stress and new cases (incidence) of work-related stress in Great Britain, 2001/2002–2010/2011

Source: Health and Safety Executive, www.hse.gov.uk/statistics/causdis/stress/index.htm (accessed 25 July 2012)

encourage other unhealthy behaviours, such as smoking, poor diet, drinking or drug taking, as ways of blunting the impact of poorly paid work for little pecuniary reward. When these are associated with problems at home, at school or with relationships, the impact can be severe.

Three main approaches to health and wellbeing have been tried: (a) from a physical health perspective – which is really insufficient to pick up the positive and negative mental health implications of work; (b) from a psychological and emotional health perspective of individuals (Danna and Griffin, 1999); or (c) from a social perspective – wellbeing is addressed by considering the implications of the outcomes of stressful work, in the effects of alcoholism, drug abuse and of other behaviours that have a wider effect on the community. The interventions we will discuss later in this chapter will reflect both the individual and collective approaches with their physical and emotional responses (see Figure 7.4).

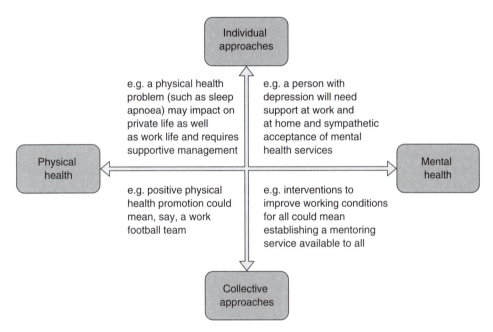

Figure 7.4   A two-by-two matrix that identifies types of interventions possible

A great deal has been written during the five or so years prior to the publication of this book. A report by the Department of Health, the Department for Work and Pensions and the Health and Safety Executive in 2005 (HM Government, 2005: 6) set out a series of objectives to achieve a society where:

- the health and wellbeing of people of working age is given the attention it deserves;
- work is recognised by all as important and beneficial, and institutional barriers to starting, returning to, or remaining in work are removed;
- health care services in the NHS and the independent sector meet the needs of people of working age so they can remain in, or ease their return to, work;

- health is not adversely affected by work, and good quality advice and support is available to, and accessible by, all;
- work offers opportunities to promote individual health and wellbeing, and access to and retention of work promotes and improves the overall health of the population;
- people with health conditions and disabilities are able to optimise work opportunities; and
- people make positive lifestyle choices from an early age and throughout their working lives.

The paper then provided a series of case studies and suggested ways in which the government would develop an improved process for the promotion of work-based wellbeing, including a stakeholder council and further consultation. In particular, the report placed an emphasis on mental health and suggested *inter alia* that there should be improved access to work-focused services to maintain affected people in meaningful community activities; provision of an extended range of services to support people in returning to work; increasing choice of evidence-based psychological therapies for people with mild to moderate depression and other mental health issues; reducing delays in receiving appropriate therapies and earlier intervention (HM Government, 2005: 21; see also Mills et al., 2007).

Professor Dame Carol Black was the National Director for Health and Work from 2005 to 2011, during which time she brought health and wellbeing to the forefront of government thinking on health and work. In 2008, she prepared a report to the government (Black, 2008) on the health of Britain's working age population and the role of healthy workplaces in promoting health and wellbeing. Following the government's response in late 2008, a set of health and wellbeing indicators were developed in 2010 as shown in Box 7.1 below.

Box 7.1   Health and Wellbeing Indicators following Black (2008)

1 Improving knowledge/perceptions about the importance of work to health and health to work

2 Improving the promotion of health and wellbeing at work

3 Reducing the incidence of work-related ill-health and injuries and their causes

4 Reducing the proportion of people out of work due to ill-health

5 Improving the self-reported health status of the working age population

6 Improving access to appropriate and timely health service support

7 Improving business productivity and performance

Whilst these are laudable, the first update report in December 2011 suggested that only two of the indicators showed any significant change, one of which was already in use: Indicator 3 shows an improving trend toward a reduction of work-related injuries (as we saw above); and Indicator 4, the gap between the employment rate of those with a long-term health condition and the overall employment rate in Britain has contracted from 12.8% at the baseline (2010) to 11.8% in the four quarters to June 2011, which may not sound much but is a statistically significant improvement from the baseline. This suggests that the emphasis on health and wellbeing at work is worth the effort, and ought to be continued. But it also suggests that much more needs to be done by government, employers, employees, trade unions, and the NHS and local authorities (CCGs and HWBs) to cement in place the gains made to date and to promote further wellbeing interventions. Although it is difficult to calculate the cost-effectiveness of interventions, the proposed opportunities cited here suggest that the interventions are not expensive, but require improved organisation to ensure they are implemented properly.

In an analysis (nef, 2012) of the first report of the health and wellbeing indicators, nef note that one of the largest contributory factors to reduced wellbeing is disability, which diminishes life satisfaction, increases anxiety and lessens overall wellbeing. Unemployed people have significantly lower wellbeing, as do people who work excessively long hours. People from black or minority ethnic groups are likely to have lower wellbeing compared to the white population. Conversely, being retired or living in rural rather than urban areas leads to higher wellbeing; nef comment that, '[A]n area's Index of Multiple Deprivation is a strong predictor of wellbeing, with crime and low income being the most important elements of deprivation' (p.3).

A national network has been established to reinforce understanding of the positive link between health and work amongst employers, employees and the general public, and involves representatives from the private sector, central and local government and the third sector. It has working groups in four areas:

1   Health and Wellbeing Local Business Partnerships – three pilots where large companies mentor local small and medium-sized enterprises (SMEs) on employee health and wellbeing.
2   Engaging SMEs – analysing the most effective ways of engaging SMEs in workplace health and wellbeing, and developing a website that brings together SME-relevant information.
3   Managing Chronic Conditions guides – developing guides for employers and employees on managing people with chronic illness in the workplace.
4   Occupational health – developing practical guidance to help occupational health services support and encourage employers in safeguarding and improving the health and wellbeing of their workforce.

More impressively, under the auspices of the European Union Programme for Employment and Social Security – PROGRESS (2007–2013), a programme on work, worklessness and health was established that has promoted an assets-based public health programme. Realising that placing an emphasis on job creation was unrealistic (although not to be forgotten), given the present recession and with austerity measures beginning to bite, the most important actions to take would include sustaining social protection and a focus on confronting workplace health-related behaviours. What this boils down to in the short term is to emphasise those aspects of an assets-based approach that may not at first sight look as though they concern employment. Redundancy, unemployment (and under-employment) and especially long-term unemployment or never having had a job are all detrimental to the individual and attack the basic needs level in the Maslow triangle (see page 9, Chapter 1 and page 17, Chapter 2). Consequently, the focus should be on early years (for all the reasons given in Chapter 6) in ways that ameliorate the worst effects of unemployment and loss of income on families; placing an emphasis on alcohol and young people; encouraging physical fitness across the life course; assisting people to improve diet and nutrition; and active labour market programmes, in particular government training programmes that are designed for personal development and are not solely to get someone into a job 'come what may'!

All these priorities should take a positive empowering approach to those out of work, assisting them to use their skills and expertise and develop wherever possible their own solutions. That does not mean abdication but a form of co-production (see Chapter 5) in which people are assisted to use their skills within a context of social protection for all. One way in which people can be helped back into work is through constructive volunteering opportunities designed to encourage personal growth and skills acquisition rather than simply using them as cheap labour. Volunteering has often assisted individuals to move from one field to another, to obtain differing experiences and to gain the necessary confidence (or rebuild lost confidence) to become employed again. Commissioners can make a huge difference by commissioning wisely, recognising the health and wellbeing benefits of purchasing social protection measures that may cost the public purse in the short term but overall have long-term savings. By understanding the situation in their local area, CCGs and HWBs have a responsibility to:

- obtain as much knowledge of the problem as possible – and to recognise that by intervening early they will save money downstream;
- build a will for change locally, by engaging leading GPs on the CCGs, local authority councillors, Directors of Public Health and public health staff, NHS and local government providers and community organisations;
- choose a method that allows everyone to become involved from the groups listed above and make the change for all in the area – don't do pilots unless it really is necessary politically – but 'go for it';
- collect data daily on the progress of the changed way of doing things. When we say daily, we mean daily – not a year after the event, but obtain data regularly in real time so that any imperfections can be ruled out quickly.[1]

By addressing psychosocial determinants of health in this way not only will the negative effects of unemployment be mitigated but a positive spirit will emerge from those who are affected. Although income is very important, it is also true that inequality is a more important predictor of poor health than income level. We should work towards encouraging 'workability' or 'employability' skills, drawing on Sen's (2002) capabilities idea – that, by empowering people to grow their own heightened capabilities, they can become resilient and develop improved coping skills. We do not need inequality to drive people to work – they want to work – but rather we need to distinguish the inherent, if unrecognised, equality of all. We should note that participation or exclusion affects long-term life chances and anything we can do to enhance inclusion will improve life chances; wages and salaries provide most families' income; exposure to hazards at work, including excessively long hours and long shift patterns are dangerous to health (the NHS is particularly prone to these features of work); and enforced part-time work has adverse social and emotional effects.

Stress at work arises from a range of imbalances: demand-control imbalances, discrepancies between effort and reward, organisational injustice, and indeed precariousness of employment (part-time working, short-term contracts, non-paid intern arrangements).[2] Self-harm is exacerbated by unemployment but can be ameliorated through effective active labour market programmes, which interestingly have the most significant impact in a model of suicide reduction, more so than family support and considerably more than the health service or unemployment benefit payments (Stuckler et al., 2009). As with other aspects of health and wellbeing, it is social connectedness that makes the difference (see Chapter 5 on community engagement); NHS and social care commissioners should enhance connectedness as a way to improve people's overall health, to create social capital and to develop co-production wherever possible.

7.2 Mental health in the workplace

Following the launch of the health and wellbeing indicators, the network described above will develop proposals for how employers can be supported to offer health-promoting activities to their employees, such as free health checks and smoking-cessation programmes; and will look at mental ill health – still one of the biggest causes of working days lost. Following the Marmot Review (2010) we can see, within a proportionate universalist approach, three levels of prevention that form a continuum:

- **Universal** interventions (for an entire working population) which will include research and action to ameliorate the factors at work that affect employees' mental health and wellbeing, such as physical (improved handling equipment, workspace organisation) and human resource (high workloads, anti-social hours), and interventions that alter job features associated with stress or anxiety or reduced wellbeing.
- **Selective** interventions for those groups of workers that appear to be at moderate to high risk, for example, those employees in specific roles where stress is part of the job, programmes to help employees manage stress, workplace counselling or schemes such as Employee Assistance Programmes (EAPs).
- **Targeted** interventions for individuals or groups that show early signs of problems, with the objective of preventing further difficulties, such as programmes to reduce the severity or longevity of symptoms, workplace counselling or mentoring, adjustments at work for people with chronic or recurring conditions to enable them to manage existing mental disorders or distress.[3]

Whilst these levels of intervention are theoretically correct there is not much good evidence of interventions that work well or are cost-effective. Seymour and Grove (2005) found 19 studies from the early 1990s to the early 2000s that included 'stress inoculation' training, development of problem solving skills, ways to reduce 'negative' survival mechanisms, identifying ways of attenuating potential stressors, CBT and other counselling techniques. There was only moderate evidence, at best, for those programmes offering universal interventions (Seymour and Grove, 2005: 22) which is perhaps unsurprising and should not detract from programmes that take a universal approach as long as these are carefully designed. Stress management may have short-term value but multi-modal approaches offered the best though limited evidence of effectiveness, particularly where improved information was associated with cognitive therapy and physical exercise.

For those who are at risk or where there are early signs of problems, there was 'strong evidence that individual approaches to stress reduction, management and prevention for a range of health care professionals was effective and preferable to multi-modal approaches' (Seymour and Grove, 2005: 23). By multi-modal we include individual and group training with a variety of differing approaches. Where multi-modal approaches provided interpersonal skills and stress management training these offered the most long lasting effects; but individually focused interventions seemed to be most effective. However, there was no evidence that social workers benefitted at all, although this was based on a very small study (Meier, 2002). Similarly there was limited evidence that physical exercise alone was effective in preventing or treating mental health problems at work (Seymour and Groves, 2005).

In the final category there was good evidence that CBT was effective for employees with common mental health problems and mental health related absenteeism (van der Klink et al., 2001; 2003; Michie and Williams, 2003; Mimura and Griffiths, 2003; Grime, 2004; Seymour and Grove, 2005). According to Yelin et al. (1996), primary care practitioners have been found to react well with patients about work-related anxiety, but this may not be universally true. Much of this bears out the results of other studies (and indeed demonstrates how careful we must be not to make assumptions about what works). For example, in one Australian study interorganisational clusters of workers or peer tutoring were found to be most effective in generating ownership and commitment of the workers (Reaveley et al., 2010), which reinforces the points above about connectedness.

7.3 Models of employee wellbeing

Employee wellbeing can be described in a number of ways. One possible model is to think about work-specific wellbeing and what can be called 'context-free' wellbeing. The first describes those aspects of the job itself that contribute to wellbeing (or often the reverse) and 'context-free' purports to describe those other aspects unrelated to work. Unfortunately nothing is 'context-free'. Contexts often merge into one another – for example, the person with incipient mental distress that is exacerbated by work. The context of home life is impacted by income and employment status. Too little income can lead to stress and undermines the supportive effects of a partner or children. A person who drinks in a social context may be doing so more frequently as a result of work pressures or it may have nothing to do with work but is the result of problematic family relationships. We must therefore specify the context, or the inter-related contexts.

Warr (1999) suggests that wellbeing can be considered on three axes: displeasure-to-pleasure, anxiety-to-comfort and depression-to-enthusiasm. Whilst we accept the importance of recognising predisposing or 'antecedent' factors in developing a model of wellbeing at work, the axes suggested by Warr (1999) are not continua or opposites. Displeasure (whatever that means) is not strictly the opposite of pleasure, unless defined specifically for those purposes; anxiety (nervousness, apprehension, disquiet) is not the opposite of comfort (which, in one dictionary definition, is correlated directly with wellbeing) other than in a very narrow sense of mental 'security'; whilst depression is not the opposite of enthusiasm. What is important here is recognising that 'health' is a broad concept and encompasses the meeting of personal preferences in socially acceptable ways, and having security of income, housing, family, and education or employment.

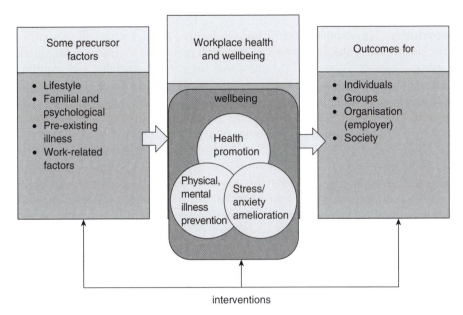

Figure 7.5 Conceptual framework for health and wellbeing at work (redrawn from Warr, 1999)

Our model of workplace health and wellbeing in Figure 7.5 draws on Warr (1999) but amends critical dimensions. First, the core model of wellbeing (in the centre of the diagram) is based on the tripartite arrangement of health promotion, illness prevention and amelioration of mental and emotional stress. Balancing these three (sets of) elements provides a dynamic approach to workplace health that at once promotes health, prevents illness and ameliorates distress. Second, the precursor factors and the outcomes are wider than Warr suggests. Because employment is such an important feature of life (especially in Western societies), people bring to their work a wide range and type of lifestyle, health or illness, age-related concerns, family difficulties and opportunities, psychological resilience and pathology, as well as matters that are directly work related such as health and safety concerns.

Employee wellbeing is thus an amalgam of these features which can be enriched or may deteriorate depending on the attitude of the employer. Good employers use their managers and HR departments to support employees, to offer mentoring and peer support, ensuring that appraisal picks up employee problems and directs employees to possibly alternative more suitable jobs; conversely, poor employers either do not have or do not care much about employee wellbeing in this holistic sense. HR departments act solely to control rather than enhance employee opportunity.

The New Economics Foundation promotes a wellbeing scale that asks many questions on five and six point scales about the way we feel; nef has promoted the five steps to wellbeing as:

- Connect ... with the people around you.
- Be active ... most importantly, discover a physical activity you enjoy.

- Take notice ... be curious.
- Keep learning ... try something new.
- Give ... do something nice for a friend or a stranger.[4]

At least one public health report has been written using these five ways to wellbeing as the analytic framework. Whilst this may appear to draw on the assets model of public health, it is really insufficient to offer a fully functioning approach to public health and health inequalities. The five ways to wellbeing are ways in which all of us can improve our wellbeing every day, by practising these behaviours regularly. From an employment perspective the five ways to wellbeing offer health, safety and welfare pointers for both employers and workers: we want staff to connect with each other in positive and supportive ways – the best companies are ones that encourage sharing, communication and involvement; good companies want staff to be and remain active for their own sake and to ensure a healthy and sustainable workforce; taking notice is essential in any work situation, encouraging staff to be curious – for example, about how to do things more efficiently or better; continuous learning and trying new activities offers rewards to the employee and the employer, whether that is formal class-based learning or, as nef constructed the idea, as a more informal way in which all workers strive to gain knowledge and self-improvement; and finally, giving to others, whether through work-based charitable donations or in a more indirect and perhaps discrete sense of offering support and assistance to those work colleagues who have a problem at a particular moment (especially, as we will see below, when someone succumbs to drug or alcohol abuse as a result of personal, familial or work-related stress).

Good workplace policies include regular policy and practice review, keeping workplace practices up to date, relevant and safe; understanding and knowing what staff think about their work, through appraisal or staff surveys; having a variety of mechanisms available for staff support, such as coaching or mentoring (for managers as well as staff); undertaking stress audits and depression or anxiety reviews, and having the resources to help anyone found to need help.[5] Good employers will use or develop diagnostic tools to support staff that may experience mental health problems, support mental health disclosure, offer mental health mediation and support, ensure there are return to work programmes and reasonable adjustments for anyone suffering a mental or serious physical illness, and adopt employee assistance programmes. As Mind suggests, developing good one-to-one relationships is often the 'single most effective development intervention [for] ... an individual'.[6]

7.4 Alcohol Abuse

Alcohol is a drug that affects a wide range of central nervous system functions. By interrelating with personality characteristics and socio-cultural expectations, it is a causal factor for intentional and unintentional injuries and harm to people other than the drinker, including reduced job performance and absenteeism, socio-economic deprivation, domestic and other forms of violence against third parties, suicide, homicide, domestic abuse, other crimes, and fatalities caused by driving or operating machinery whilst under the influence of alcohol. Alcohol abuse contributes to risky sexual behaviour; leads to low foetal birth-weight, cognitive deficiencies and foetal alcohol disorders; is addictive; and is an immunosuppressant, increasing the risk of communicable diseases including tuberculosis. Alcohol is a carcinogen and increases the risk of cancers of the mouth and pharynx, oesophagus, stomach, colon, rectum and breast. Finally, alcohol is linked with CHD: it would appear to be cardio-protective in low doses but there is some doubt about this. However, at higher doses it can lead to serious clinical problems (Anderson et al., 2009).

In England, 38% of men and 16% of women aged 16 to 64 years have an alcohol use disorder, which is equivalent to approximately 8.2 million people (DH, 2004). This stark statistic lies behind many of the attempts to tackle problem drinking. Up to 2.6 million children live with parents who drink at 'hazardous' levels and around 700,000 children are thought to live with dependent drinkers.[7] Turning Point highlights Joseph Rowntree Foundation funded research which found that children who see their parents drunk are twice as likely to get drunk themselves. Deaths from the toxic effects of alcohol are increasing steadily in the United Kingdom. Alcohol-related mortality rates are higher in men and increase with age, generally reaching highest levels in middle-aged adults. In one study the 45–64 year age group included roughly 25% of the total UK population but was responsible for half of all alcohol-related deaths (Erskine et al., 2010). More importantly there was an association between alcohol-related mortality and socio-economic deprivation, with higher rates in more deprived areas, with higher mortality in urban compared to rural areas, the differences remaining after adjustment for socio-economic deprivation (Erskine et al., 2010).

Tackling what can only be described as a crisis has challenged and continues to elude all administrations. A number of papers have been written over the last ten years on pricing mechanisms and ways of using cost to restrict alcohol sales. Unfortunately there are a number of barriers to action. The price elasticity of demand for alcohol products is less than one (i.e. it is *inelastic*): that is, changes in price have a relatively small effect on the quantity of alcohol consumed (see, for example, Purshouse et al., 2009); supermarkets and other retailers are not keen to lose business; and alcohol use is so deeply entrenched in society that reducing consumption is fraught with wider complications. Even government action to place a minimum cost per unit is unlikely to have an effect. Recent government action on binge drinking of alcohol focuses heavily on tackling the availability of cheap alcohol through the introduction of a minimum unit price for alcohol and consulting on a ban on multi-buy promotions in the off licence trade. The government is committed to reducing irresponsible promotions in pubs and clubs, developing alcohol anti-fraud measures, stopping unacceptable marketing and advertising, and developing a scheme to verify people's ages, which will apply to alcohol company websites and associated social media (Secretary of State for Health, 2012). However, setting a minimum per unit price for alcohol creates a number of complications: to be effective the price per unit needs to be high – probably well above 50p, but that will penalise those who drink sensibly or do not drink large amounts.

Similarly, a briefing in 2012 for Police and Crime Commissioner candidates was understandably concerned with advising them to take an active role in licensing decisions; campaign for minimum pricing; ensure tougher enforcement of alcohol free zones, under age sales and serving people when drunk; prioritise drink driving campaigns and clampdowns; and use budgets to invest in alcohol treatment services and signpost offenders (e.g. cautioned) to alcohol treatment services, through liaison with A&E.[8]

Although some of the policies advocated by the Alcohol Policy website will assist in tackling problem drinking, there is too little in the government's strategy or alternative policy advice that is concerned with early preventive mechanisms, primary and secondary school programmes, intervening in domestic situations likely to encourage drinking, and bringing the implications of alcohol related problems to the attention of young people and young adults before the problems becomes acute. Alcohol use (and abuse) is so endemic that we fail to see the effects on domestic violence, street brawls particularly on Friday and Saturday nights, old people drinking alone at home or the well-to-do pensioner who starts drinking by 11.00 every morning and is more or less comatose by early evening. However, we see again the importance of intervening early. By improving childhood experiences we will see significant improvement 10 or 15 years down the line. Perhaps that is too long for many commissioners; but if we had done this in the mid-1990s we would be seeing the benefits now.

Resources for dealing with excessive alcohol consumption are nonetheless available. Brief interventions have been shown by a meta-analysis to reduce all-cause mortality by about 50% (Cuijpers et al., 2004). The impact of such a target would depend largely on who is defined as a 'problem drinker', their excess morbidity and mortality in the absence of treatment or other intervention, implementation fidelity, the proportion not already treated and the degree of targeting. Four research papers were included in the meta-analysis, of which one is very old and two were variants of research on cardiovascular disease (Chick et al., 1985; Fleming et al., 1999; Wutzke et al., 2002). If the literature is interpreted to mean 'harmful' drinkers rather than 'dependent' drinkers then using the prevalence figures for the area in question and the calculated relative risk of all-cause mortality, the population attributable fractions[9] can be assessed. By and large the reduction in all-cause mortality from brief interventions is between 5% and 6% for men and between 3% and 4% for women. This equates approximately to a sixth of all deaths per annum for females and a quarter for men in the 45–64 age range – a target worth aiming for from just one of the treatment options available.

A more recent meta-analysis of the effectiveness of brief interventions for harmful alcohol consumption noted a positive effect of brief interventions on alcohol consumption, mortality, morbidity, alcohol-related injuries, alcohol-related social consequences, health care resource use, and laboratory indicators of harmful alcohol use (Kaner et al., 2007). A systematic review of 12 studies indicated that a combination of educational and clinical support programmes increased screening and advice providing rates of GPs and primary health care providers from 32% to 45% (Anderson et al., 2004). Other opportunities to reduce drinking include school programmes to tackle drug and alcohol misuse, offering alternative outlets for young people's energies, suggesting voluntary work for isolated elderly people, and working with abusing families on strategies to address misogynistic control and anger management. Cognitive behavioural therapies for alcohol dependence have been developed and one systematic review of 17 papers on behavioural self-control training found a quite reasonable combined effect size of 0.33 for reduced alcohol consumption and alcohol-related difficulties (Walters, 2000). Other programmes have been less successful and have not led to sustained effects on behaviour (Jones et al., 2007). On the other hand some social marketing programmes appear to have had valuable effects in the short term (up to 12 months) and two studies have reported longer-term improvements (Stead et al., 2007).

Studies of domestic abuse frequently report high rates of alcohol and other drug involvement that is known to impair judgement, reduce inhibition and increase aggression.[10] At face value it is hard to argue with the figures. In the USA, 92% of domestic abuse perpetrators reported use of alcohol or other drugs on the day of the assault (Brookoff et al., 1997) and in another study the percentage of perpetrators under the influence of alcohol when they assault their partners ranged from 48% to 87%. The odds of any male-to-female physical aggression are eight times higher on days when the perpetrators drink alcohol than on days with no alcohol consumption, with the chances of severe male-to-female physical aggression on drinking days more than 11 times higher (Fals-Stewart, 2003). However, there is little research to indicate that alcohol *causes* domestic violence. Although amongst men who drink heavily there is a higher rate of assaults resulting in injury, the majority of men classified as high-level drinkers do not abuse their partners. Also, the majority (76%) of physically abusive incidents occur in the absence of alcohol use.[11]

Violence against women is a major criminal, social and public health concern and contributes to high levels of morbidity and mortality. In one study of gender-based violence in the United States, 17% of women reported rape or attempted rape, and more than one-fifth of women reported domestic violence, stalking or both. There is now strong evidence that these forms of violence lead to mental illness and psychosocial problems. Given the description of alcohol use, abuse and dependence, it is evident that wellbeing is compromised when alcohol is consumed in excess, not only by the person who abuses alcohol but also by friends, family and workmates. The answer to the points made above is health promotion and early (primary) prevention. This will not be easy but the way forward may be to link alcohol use strategies with other health and social care activities that offer a complementary set of motivations and thus have a multiplier effect.

7.5 Conclusion

Workplace wellbeing is extremely important for all adults. Ensuring positive mental health from the age of 18 to 68 or older (a full 50 years of life, which for most people in work means something around 60% of their life) means intervening to offer both health promoting interventions and interventions to assist those who have mental health problems at work. These may be either caused by work or as a result of personal lives outside work but which have an influence on work behaviours. There is a lot that can be done, some by employers and some by public and independent agencies. In particular screening for depression and other mental health problems at work is important, whilst health promoting activities and preventive strategies will ensure that most people remain healthy. Reducing stress in the workplace is a critical activity as is ensuring that an individual is given just sufficient stimulation and stretching targets without going too far and overloading their abilities. Linking alcohol abuse and worklessness could become an important preventive strategy.

However, alcohol abuse needs to be the focus of preventive strategies as it is a major contributor to poor health, risky health behaviours and violence towards others, including domestic abuse, all of which have far-reaching implications. We have highlighted the evidence for brief interventions, concluding that approaches to the prevention of alcohol abuse need to go beyond this and require structural changes and social marketing to promote responsible drinking and an awareness of the harms of alcohol abuse. Alongside this, a commitment to prevention and early identification needs to be operationalised within mainstream services, particularly primary care. CCCGs and HWBS are well positioned to realise this.

Notes

1 These points were made in a powerful presentation by Sir Harry Burns, CMO Scottish Government, at a conference entitled, EU PROGRESS Project: Working for Equity in Health, held in Brussels on 26 November 2012, organised by HAPI (the Health Action Partnership International) and the Scottish Government, funded by the EU PROGRESS programme.

2 Peter Goldblatt, speaking at the same conference.

3 Source: www.bohrf.org.uk/downloads/cmh_rev.pdf (accessed 20 March 2013).

4 'Five ways to wellbeing', www.neweconomics.org/projects/five-ways-well-being (accessed 25 July 2012).

5 See, for example, Mind Workplace, www.mind.org.uk/workplace (accessed 20 August 2012).

6 www.mind.org.uk/workplace (accessed 20 August 2012).

7 For a longer discussion, see a note on Turning Point at www.alcoholpolicy.net/domestic_violence (accessed 20 August 2012).

8 www.alcoholpolicy.net (accessed 20 August 2012).

9 The contribution of a risk factor to a disease (or death) is quantified using the population attributable fraction (PAF). PAF is the proportional reduction in population disease or mortality that would occur if exposure to a risk factor were reduced to an alternative ideal exposure scenario (e.g. from some tobacco use to no tobacco use). Many diseases are caused by multiple risk factors, and individual risk factors may interact in their impact on overall risk of disease. As a result, PAFs for individual risk factors often overlap and add up to more than 100%.

10 About.com, at http://alcoholism.about.com/cs/abuse/a/aa990331.htm (accessed 20 August 2012).

11 About.com, at http://alcoholism.about.com/cs/abuse/a/aa990331.htm (accessed 20 August 2012).

CHAPTER 8

Depression, Diabetes, Dementia

This chapter considers the inter-relationship between depression, diabetes and dementia. Although there is firm evidence that these three conditions are related, little has been done by commissioners or providers to make the links explicit. Our contention is that services should ensure that (a) depression is always correctly identified and treated, however minor; (b) diabetes (especially Type 2 diabetes) should be considered a disease that as much reflects early years support (or the lack of effective care during the early years) as the effects of lifestyle choices later; and (c) the repercussions of diabetes, especially micro-angiopathy, are implicated in the incidence and prevalence of dementia in some patients. Other related conditions are also considered including cerebrovascular and cardiovascular disease.

8.1 Introduction

Although a great deal has been known about the detailed aetiology of diabetes for at least 30 years, the incidence and prevalence of diabetes continues to increase. During the last decade real progress has been made in understanding the genetic epidemiology, the medical and social prognosis and methods of prevention. In particular the incidence and prevalence of Type 2 diabetes can be delayed and possibly prevented, but this will require a sea-change in public attitudes towards nutrition, exercise and more healthy lifestyles (Elasy, 2010) and a transformation in health care provision.

One possibility that may make diabetes prevention at once more acceptable but more disturbing is the confluence of knowledge about depression, diabetes and dementia, which together with other medical conditions, notably oral health, obesity, dyslipidaemia and (lack of) exercise create both an alarming but ultimately powerful encouragement to accept advice and change lifestyle. This chapter will look at these subjects together, at least to the extent that they have common features or are precursors for one another. Many wellbeing interventions are common to these conditions, or are closely related. Another group of conditions that have genetic markers in common are diabetes, Alzheimer's disease (dementia), Parkinson's disease, multiple sclerosis and rheumatoid arthritis. We shall review the evidence and suggest cost-effective health promotion and preventive measures. Finally, depression is associated with coronary heart disease and cerebrovascular disease and we will consider briefly the health and wellbeing interventions that can reduce the consequences of CHD and CVD.

8.2 Aetiology and prevalence of diabetes

Diabetes mellitus is one of the commonest chronic and disabling conditions worldwide. Both incidence and prevalence are increasing internationally, largely as a result of unhealthy lifestyles (poor diet and nutrition and lack of exercise). The UK prevalence of diabetes in the adult population is 4.45% with England having the highest prevalence at 5.5%. Type 2 diabetes usually appears in middle-aged or older people, although it is being diagnosed in younger people more frequently and it is known to affect South Asian people at a younger age (Tuomilehto at al., 2001). In England, the prevalence for people aged over 55 reaches 11% for men and 8% for women, increasing to over 15% for men and over 13% for women above age 65 (Diabetes UK, 2010); 90% of adult diabetes is Type 2, whereas for children and adolescents the figure is the reverse with over 97% having Type 1 diabetes. However, this figure masks the rapidly increasing numbers of adolescents with Type 2 diabetes largely as a result of obesity.

The disease is characterised by chronic hyperglycaemia,[1] which can cause macro-vascular problems, such as myocardial infarction (heart attack), cerebrovascular disease, peripheral vascular disease and stroke; and micro-vascular disorders, such as renal disease (nephropathy[2]), retinopathy,[3] microangiopathy[4] (especially in the brain) and neuropathy.[5] These may all be present in people with undiagnosed diabetes or pre-diabetes, and various risk factors for depression (smoking, lack of exercise, dietary habits, obesity and co-morbid cardiovascular complications) are also common in undiagnosed diabetes or pre-diabetes.

Type 1 diabetes is an autoimmune disease that manifests in childhood and late adolescence, in which complete insulin deficiency[6] leads to severe complications if untreated. Self-care is an essential part of diabetes management (giving insulin injections, taking oral medication, maintaining a specific diet, weight loss, blood pressure management) and is not done well in up to 50% of patients. Even with intensive therapy, blood glucose levels rise by around 15% over 15 years (compared to a rise of more than 20% with conventional care) but weight gain can be as high as 10 pounds (up to 5kg) over the same period (in contrast to conventional therapy which is only half that amount).[7]

A great deal of research has been done over the last 20 to 30 years on prevention of Type 2 diabetes. Lifestyle interventions (weight loss, exercise, etc.), especially those that take a comprehensive approach to correcting several lifestyle factors simultaneously (Tuomilehto et al., 2001) appear to be at least as effective as pharmacological interventions (excluding herbal remedies that are not statistically significant) in delaying progress towards Type 2 diabetes in patients with impaired glucose tolerance (Gillies et al., 2007). Interventions to improve self-care may thus lead to more cost-effective use of medicines (Cobden et al., 2010).

Unsurprisingly, very strong associations exist between patient behaviours, attitudes towards self-care, health outcomes and cost in Type 2 diabetes. Although medication adherence is well researched and may influence diabetic outcomes, cardiovascular risk, mortality rates and health care resource usage, such as GP time or bed usage in hospitals (not to mention the impact on depression and dementia discussed below), these factors are rarely seen within cost calculations (Cobden et al., 2010). In Chapter 10 we will consider the generalised cost-effectiveness of interventions in more detail. In practice, control of CVD risk factors, such as glycaemia, hypertension and dyslipidaemia, are poorly done despite all the evidence, which makes diabetes prevention an attractive prospect to those concerned with CVD and CHD (Karam and McFarlane, 2011). In older adults 90% of all new cases of diabetes are attributable to five risk factors – physical activity level, diet, smoking, alcohol habits and obesity (Mozaffarian et al., 2009).

Commissioning groups will be required to incorporate NICE quality standards into their plans across one or more domains of the Outcomes Framework[8] which will provide a read-across between domains (MSD, 2013). MSD[9] suggest that this will ensure that Domain 1 (preventing premature death) will link with improvements in under-75 mortality rate from cardiovascular disease; and Domain 2 (enhancing quality of life for people with long-term conditions) will link with the importance of ensuring people feel supported to manage their own condition (MSD, 2013: 4). Self-management is a critical area for diabetic care and there has been too little research on what interventions work best in improving self-care. Although the 13 NICE quality standards recognise the importance of education and good clinician–patient engagement, unfortunately there is too little emphasis on self-management and the reasons many patients do not actively self-manage their weight, nutrition, diet and exercise (NICE, 2011).

8.3 Diabetes and depression

The incidence and prevalence of depression associated with Type 2 diabetes poses a question of causation. Do people become depressed as a result of their diabetes, as may happen with any chronic disease? Is their lifestyle, diet, nutrition and exercise regime a manifestation of depression which leads to the development of diabetes? Or are the two linked in some other way, perhaps in complex genetic interactions? Depression in patients with diabetes is associated with a higher burden of medical symptoms such as hyperglycaemia, diabetic complications (Rustad et al., 2011), additional functional impairment, poor self-care (adherence to diet, exercise, cessation of smoking, and medications), increased cardiac risk factors, increased vascular complications and higher mortality (Katon et al., 2006; Cobden et al., 2010).

Both depression and diabetes contribute significantly to the global burden of disease. A recent meta-analysis demonstrated an association between both mild and severe depressive disorders and diabetes (Eaton et al., 1996; Mezuk et al., 2008). It would appear there is a relationship both ways, a two-way street that seems difficult to navigate (Renn et al., 2011); there is a well-established link between depression and an increased risk for diabetes, but diabetes (Wu et al., 2011) is also a moderate risk factor for depression, which increases considerably with complications to around a three-fold increased risk of depression (de Groot et al., 2012). This is perhaps unsurprising as depression is associated with severe obesity, one of the key risk factors for diabetes (Onyike et al., 2003), as are lack of physical exercise and poor self-care. The population attributable risk of diabetes from depression is of the order of 7% to 9% using diagnostic interviews (Mezuk et al., 2008; Campayo et al., 2010), but 26% using depressive symptoms self-reported scores (Ismail, 2009).

Depression is associated with a 37% increased risk of subsequent diabetes mainly in Type 2 disease (Knol et al., 2006). Treating depression with antidepressants may increase diabetes risk by as much as two-fold following moderate to high usage for over 24 months (Andersohn et al., 2009) although it is unclear whether this is an independent effect (Campayo et al., 2010). Andersohn et al.'s paper somewhat overstates the effects of antidepressant medication as only one tricyclic (out of eight reviewed) and two SSRIs (out of six reviewed) and none of the other medications considered were associated in a statistically significant way with an increased rate of diabetes. Untreated depression, including mild forms of the disorder, is associated with a higher incidence of diabetes. Depression and diabetes lead to less physical activity, smoking, unhealthy diet and poorer adherence to treatment (Gonsalez et al., 2007). There is some evidence that the prevalence of anxiety disorders and eating disorders are increased in diabetes (Ismail, 2009). Risk factors for depression are shown in Box 8.1.

Box 8.1   Risk Factors for Depression

- Family members, especially biological relatives, or friends who have been depressed.

- Use and abuse of alcohol, nicotine or illicit drugs.

- Female gender.

- Traumatic childhood experiences.

- Psychosocial hazards and/or disadvantage, e.g. unemployment, poor housing, lack of citizenship.

- Stressful life events, such as the death of a loved one, or significant stress at work.

- Social exclusion or loneliness, and having few friends or other personal relationships.

- Recently having given birth (PPD).

- Having been depressed previously.

- Serious illness, such as cancer, diabetes, heart disease, Alzheimer's or HIV/AIDS.

- Low self-esteem and/or a predisposition to being overly dependent, self-critical or pessimistic.

- Taking certain high blood pressure medications, sleeping pills or certain other medications.

In addition to these factors there are psychosocial phenomena. Being a woman, for example, in many societies, increases the chances of depression over that of men, largely as a result of material conditions, deprivation, being a single parent, together with the micro-discriminations in society and the lack of power and personal control. Alongside this, the social construction of depression disadvantages women over men (Busfield, 1996). All of these could be implicated in the incidence of depression. A common genetic, biological or environmental origin for depression and Type 2 diabetes is also a possibility. Six hypotheses have been advanced:

- shared environmental and genetic development factors (see above);
- dopamine reward systems are linked to both obesity and impulsive disorders;

- a direct link exists through diet, weight, lack of exercise and smoking;
- increased activity of the hypothalamic-pituitary-adrenal system increases cortisol and cat-echolamine;
- inflammatory factors involved in the causal pathway to insulin resistance may be increased in depression;
- hyperglycaemia may activate the sympathetic nervous system and may lead to micro-vascular cerebrovascular disease (and thus to dementia as well). (Ismail, 2009)

Each of these hypotheses is theoretical and somewhat conjectural, and further research is needed to understand better the aetiology and prognosis of depression and diabetes, linked with other conditions, notably dementia. It is likely that we will find a number of genetic, environmental components common on the causative pathway of the diseases, and we should be on the look-out for more holistic approaches (Ismail, 2009).

8.4 Interventions to prevent or ameliorate depression and diabetes

Given the self-reinforcing, systemic nature of the disorders, and the significant intercon-nection of the symptoms of depression and diabetes, we need to consider carefully the interventions that are needed to tackle the burden of disease, and more importantly to prevent the disease occurring and to ameliorate its early consequences. Narayan et al. (2012) have called for a paradigm shift in Type 2 diabetes prevention and control through evidence-based and cost-effective primary and secondary prevention of Type 2 disease. They suggest four policy changes are required:

- integrating primary and secondary prevention along a clinical continuum;
- recognising the central importance of early detection of pre-diabetes and undiagnosed diabe-tes in implementing cost-effective prevention and control;
- integrating community and clinical expertise, and resources, within organised and affordable service delivery systems; and
- sharing and adopting evidence-based policies at the global level.

Whilst Narayan et al. (2012) are concerned almost solely with diabetes, given the preced-ing discussion of depression and diabetes, their recommendations underline the impor-tance of achieving an integrated community-led approach to clinical care that places an emphasis on primary and secondary prevention bringing together mental health care, diabetes care and (as we will see later in the chapter) care for older people, and dementia care (with a number of other specialty inputs to reduce further the overall burden of disease). As we have seen, mild to moderate depression is a risk factor for diabetes, and diabetes is a risk factor for depression.

Table 8.1 suggests a wide range of primary and secondary preventive measures for averting or at least controlling the complications of diabetes and depression (and which may have implications for dementia). The two rows enclosed in a bold border are the areas that could form the basis of a collaborative primary-community integrated service that brings diabetes and depression (mental health) care together, linked where possible to dementia care, smoking cessation and weight and exercise programmes. This ideally

Table 8.1   Treating depression and diabetes together

Primary Prevention of Diabetes[10]	Primary Prevention of Depression[11]	Secondary Prevention of Diabetes	Secondary Prevention of Depression
Screening for pre-diabetes	Screening for depression in those with pre-diabetes or diabetes	Screening for undiagnosed Type 2 diabetes	Screening and treatment for mild to moderate depression
Intensive lifestyle intervention – weight loss, exercise, nutrition, self-care	Lifestyle intervention targeting weight loss, exercise, smoking cessation	Glycaemic control	Training in coping skills, social problem solving, social skills, communication skills and (where necessary) parenting
Provide detailed but understandable information on the effects of pre-diabetes	Offer information sessions to patients and carers	Provide detailed but understandable information on the effects of diabetes	
Possible use of oral pharmacology where indicated	Low-intensity psychosocial interventions, psychological interventions, medication and referral for further assessment and interventions[12]	Self-monitoring of blood sugar levels	Medication, high-intensity psychological interventions, combined treatments, collaborative care and referral for further assessment and interventions[13]
Ensure blood glucose monitoring in asymptomatic patients		Blood pressure and lipid controls	
Smoking cessation counselling	Tackle wider social problems (housing, crime, employment, schooling)	Comprehensive food care	

should be established around the needs of individual patients and service users so that a truly person-centred approach to care is developed, with 'personal shoppers' (care workers or volunteers) supporting service users in order to tackle their lack of interest in, or compliance with, or genuine inability to provide self-monitoring and self-care. An excellent report in 2010 from a working group established by Diabetes UK and the NHS (Diabetes UK, 2010) offers assistance on emotional and psychological support and care in diabetes, and recognises the need for mental health and diabetic care to be provided together. One of the main objectives of the working group's remit was to, '[I]dentify competences for people with diabetes and to those providing emotional and psychological support to facilitate optimal self care' (Diabetes UK, 2010: 9).

Whilst Narayan et al. are undoubtedly right, it is worth noting that by intervening in the early years to improve parenting skills and child support (see Chapter 6) we can influence the longer-term life chances of those who might otherwise go on to develop diabetes. Some Type 2 diabetes occurs as a result of natural events, such as pregnancy; but in the main, as we have seen, the main risk factors are diet, lack of exercise, obesity and poor self-management. These can be ameliorated well before the likely incidence of disease. By taking an assets-based approach we can engage the positive opportunities that individuals, families and communities can bring to bear. Instead of a pathological mental framework we need a 'salutogenic' framework in which we focus on what people can do rather than what they cannot. Some recent writers have drawn attention to ways of empowering patients to take responsibility for self-management in ways that are acceptable to them. By engaging patients in a genuine dialogue about their lifestyles, resources and needs, empowered patients have improved their own self-care markedly. Not only is this good for patients but it is cost effective (Simon et al., 2007).

From this perspective, lifestyle interventions such as exercise on prescription assist in improving general health as well as offering benefits for those at risk of Type 2 diabetes. 'Diabetes-specific quality of life, general health-related quality of life, and social support… increased', as a result of regular exercise, and participants 'reported improvements in their overall diabetes-related health… and improved self management' (de Groot et al., 2012: 164). A combination approach of exercise and CBT in both depression and diabetes outcomes provides an opportunity to achieve improvements in both at the same time, and 'exercise can be used to achieve multiple benefits for adults with Type 2 diabetes' (de Groot et al., 2012: 157).

8.5 Depression, diabetes and dementia

Evidence of a connection between depression, diabetes and dementia has been available for a long time, but the preceding ten years or so has seen much greater interest from researchers. This has been driven by a range of factors. In part it is due to the rapid increase in the prevalence of Type 2 diabetes which has demanded a response from governments, health agencies and professional staff; in part it is due to the development of better quality mental health services largely based on community treatment and support models; and in part because of the explosion of gene studies, especially single nucleotide polymorphisms (SNP) analysis that following the mapping of the human genome, notably Genome Wide Association Studies (GWAS) and interactome methodologies.

Of those risk factors for dementia (diabetes, hypertension, dyslipidaemia and obesity) diabetes and obesity have shown the most consistent association (Kloppenburg et al., 2008). For example, one study, admittedly with a relatively small sample, found not only an association between diabetes and mild cognitive impairment (MCI) and dementia (mostly Alzheimer's disease) but also the risk of progression to dementia (Velayudhan et al., 2010). People with diabetes had up to a 1.5 fold greater change in cognitive function than those without diabetes; people with diabetes have both a larger deterioration in cognitive function and a greater risk of cognitive decline (Cukierman et al., 2005).

One possible explanation is the effects of chronic hyperglycaemia that may cause brain micro-angiopathy probably due to similar mechanisms to those occurring in retinopathy and other micro-vascular complications (Bourdel-Marchasson et al., 2010). Diabetes and pre-diabetes (elevated adiposity and hyperinsulinemia) are related to a higher risk of

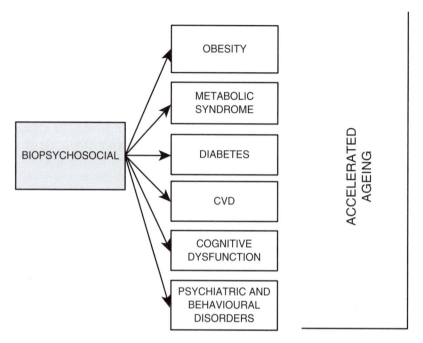

Figure 8.1   Interconnections between diabetes and other functional disorders (reproduced by permission of Dr Shahrad Taheri, University of Birmingham)

dementia, including late onset Alzheimer's disease (LOAD) although the associations are stronger for vascular dementia than LOAD (Luchsinger, 2010). This suggests that strategies to prevent Type 2 diabetes may work in preventing dementia.

The classical and genetic epidemiology of these diseases is challenging. Obesity, diabetes, dementia and depression are separately complex diseases. Although a large literature exists on the association between diabetes and dementia there is less, although growing, on the cross-relationships between the others. One study found that levels of HbA1c, a key marker of glycaemic control, were not related to dementia per se but to the incidence of severe cognitive impairment (Brayne et al., 2005) (although the authors warn of the bias and confounders faced by epidemiological studies in this complex area). However, diabetes and pre-diabetes accelerate the progression from MCI to dementia, and anticipate dementia occurrence by more than three years in people with MCI (on a Kaplan-Meier survival analysis) (Xu et al., 2010).

An innovative approach to genetic understanding of these disorders is to compare GWAS that reveal common variants (such as SNPs) that predispose to complex human diseases, with the interactomes[14] that demonstrate the molecular reality hosting the susceptibility genes. A study of five neurodegenerative and autoimmune complex disorders (Parkinson's disease, Alzheimer's disease, multiple sclerosis, rheumatoid arthritis, and Type 1 diabetes) demonstrated both immune function information and genetic links between the five disorders. In particular there was a strong association between Type 1 diabetes and Alzheimer's disease (Menon and Farina, 2011).

Genetic susceptibility may be driven by variations in some common genes, either the same variant may confer susceptibility to distinct diseases or different variants in the same gene predispose to distinct diseases. However, the inclusion of Alzheimer's disease suggests both an immunological and an inflammatory contribution. Given that regular use of anti-inflammatory drugs reduces the odds of developing Alzheimer's disease (and there is an established association between Type 2 diabetes and cognitive decline and dementia) there is the possibility of a preventive strategy that targets the three disorders simultaneously, and we might add supports both health (in generating additional healthy life years) and wellbeing both in those with the disorder and their carers.

8.6 Association between diabetes, cardiovascular disease and cerebrovascular disease

Depression and diabetes are also associated with cerebrovascular and cardiovascular disease. In part this is due to common aetiological factors, but in part to mostly unexplained factors. If unmanaged or poorly managed, diabetes can lead to very serious medical complications including limb amputation, advanced periodontal disease, blindness, neuropathy, cerebrovascular disease, kidney failure and premature death (Renn et al., 2011). Despite evidence that glycaemic control, as well as that of other CVD risk factors such as hypertension, decreases morbidity and mortality in those with diabetes, control of glycaemia and other CVD risk factors remains generally worse than it should be. This makes the idea of diabetes prevention attractive in order to control the risk of CVD, given that the risk is increasing in those with pre-diabetes (Karam and McFarlane, 2011). Meta-analyses of available trials show that all major antihypertensive drugs protect against cardiovascular complications, probably because of the by-product effect of lowering blood pressure (Perk et al., 2012). Intensive management of hyperglycaemia in diabetes and intensive treatment of blood pressure reduce the risk of micro-vascular complications and to some extent cardiovascular disease (Perk et al., 2012: 1680).

These facts suggest that diabetes treatment should be given as assertively as is reasonable, largely because of the varied and extensive secondary effects of the disease. Multimodal behavioural interventions should be developed that integrate health education, physical exercise and psychological therapies, and that where clinically significant symptoms of depression or anxiety are evident psychotherapy or medication should be considered (Perk et al., 2012: 1671). Multiple interventions including CBT, specialised health care and social care professionals, with exercise training and stress management, will help to achieve a healthier lifestyle with concomitant benefits.

a) Association between depression and cardiovascular disease

Depression in patients with coronary heart disease is common. The point prevalence for patients with a recent heart attack (myocardial infarction – MI) or unstable angina (acute coronary syndrome – ACS) and elevated depressive symptoms is between 17% and 46% (Davidson, 2011). Almost 40% of CHD patients have clinically significant depression and major depressive disorders are estimated to occur in almost one tenth of CHD patients. All-cause mortality almost doubles where patients have depression and CHD. Depression in CHD patients is associated with lowered quality of life, and, of all the predictors of the quality of life one year after a heart attack, depression was the most important.

Depression in post-acute angina patients is associated with high medical costs, reduced ability to undertake work and lost productive activity. As Davidson (2011) notes, patients with a chronic medical condition, such as CHD, and comorbid depression have significantly more out-patient appointments, A&E attendances, days off work and related disabilities. Clinical depression (relative risk (RR): 2.69) confers a higher risk of CHD than the 'traditional' risk factors: hypertension (RR: 1.92), smoking (RR: 1.71), or diabetes (RR: 1.47) (figures given in Blumenthal, 2007, reproduced from Rozanski et al., 2005). The conclusion of Blumenthal's study is that exercise is the most significant intervention for both depression *and* CHD. Many NHS commissioners would be well advised to pay for exercise on prescription for such patients (on the understanding that patients undertook to do the exercise fully and regularly!). In another study, the concurrence of diabetes and depression was associated with a significantly increased risk of death from all causes, beyond that from having either diabetes or depression alone. Hazard ratios for all-cause mortality with depression alone were 1.2, with diabetes alone, 1.88, and with depression and diabetes together, 2.5. For CHD mortality the hazard ratios were raised a little by the presence of depression or diabetes but were not statistically significant (Egede et al., 2005).

There is little clear agreement on why depression and CHD are related, although there is some evidence that assertive treatment of depression reduces the likelihood of a cardiac event very slightly. As Frasure-Smith and Lesperance (2005: Abstract p. 39) suggest: 'While debate continues about the causal relationship between CHD and depression, the best treatment strategy to improve prognosis in depressed CHD patients remains intensive modification of standard CHD risk factors in combination with treatment of depression to improve life quality'. Almost certainly the most effective preventive measures are first to encourage people to stop smoking, which should continue to be the strategy for commissioning health and wellbeing in this disease area, and second, to encourage exercise. Self-reported depression using a standardised questionnaire and clinical markers of mild to severe depression have been shown to be associated with an increased risk for CHD, but there was no clear evidence that depression is a risk factor for CVD (Nabi et al., 2010).

Research suggests that positive psychological wellbeing (PPW) is associated with cardiovascular health, although a lot of the research to date has involved older people and has not identified the ways in which psychological wellbeing affects cardiovascular disease (or vice versa). In a study that investigated the association between two aspects of wellbeing (emotional vitality and optimism) and three definitions of CHD, positive psychological wellbeing was associated with reduced risk of CHD (Boehm et al., 2011). For every unit increase in PPW there was a modest (10% to 25%) but consistent reduction in the risk of a coronary event, which the authors suggest is consistent with previous research (e.g. Giltay et al., 2006; Kubzansky and Thurston, 2007). Whether the results are generalisable is open to doubt as the sample was relatively healthy and did not include 'blue collar' workers or unemployed people. On the other hand it was a large sample (almost 8,000 people) without a prior cardiovascular event (fatal CHD, first non-fatal myocardial infarction or first definite angina) and had broadly similar groups of men and women. Similarly, Arbelaez et al. (2007), when studying the incidence of stroke in a cohort of 5,525 elderly men and women aged 65 and older (who were prospectively followed from 1989 to 2000 as participants in a Cardiovascular Health Study), found that worse depressive symptoms were associated with the risk of ischemic stroke but that inflammation (as an indicator) appeared not to modify the results.

b) Depression associated with other physical disorders

Unsurprisingly, depression is associated with many physical disorders. Cancer, for example, is often associated with depression, which is probably an adaptive response and appears to affect men and women equally despite higher rates of depression in women without other morbidities, 'usually as a result of intrinsic biological or psychological vulnerabilities … [or] … disproportionate exposure to stressful events and circumstances' (Miller et al., 2011c: 959). Parkinson's disease and other neurological conditions provide alternative examples. Roughly 40% of people with Parkinson's disease will suffer from an episode of depression, which is often missed because some of the symptoms of PD are similar to those of depression.[15] Reduced speech and slow movements both occur in depression and Parkinson's disease. The aetiology is unclear, as living with PD is for some people inherently depressing, but there may also be direct neurological effects. Another disease in which depression is more likely is multiple sclerosis. Again, whether depression arises from the neurological effects of the disease or the degree to which the implications of the disability lead to depression is unclear. There is growing evidence that cognitive symptoms may be more widespread than was once believed (MS Society, 2012) and that treating the symptoms of depression can have both positive and negative effects (Hart et al., 2005). Focusing on the efficacy of exercise interventions enhances wellbeing (McAuley et al., 2007); and by offering tailored home visits for mental health assessment, with an outpatient clinic co-managed with a neuro-psychiatrist, and a CBT clinic, MS patients have shown wellbeing improvements (Askey-Jones et al., 2009).

This group of neurological disorders are prime candidates for improvements in health and wellbeing from a preventive or health promotion viewpoint. For instance, NICE recommends that people with PD should have specialist nurse input to support patients and carers, to aid communication (NICE, 2006) and provide higher levels of physiotherapy. Particular consideration should include gait re-education, improvement of balance and flexibility; enhancement of aerobic capacity; improvement of movement initiation; improvement of functional independence, including mobility and activities of daily living, and provision of advice regarding safety in the home environment. Many of these interventions are provided now but not on a consistent or equitable basis. All these interventions will improve wellbeing by enabling better quality movement, although a recent report suggested that the benefits are only short term; a large, well designed, randomised controlled trial is needed to assess the efficacy and cost-effectiveness of physiotherapy for treating PD in the longer term (Tomlinson et al., 2012). In addition, Alexander Technique therapy may be beneficial to patients with PD by 'helping them to make lifestyle adjustments that affect both the physical nature of the condition and the person's attitudes to having PD' (NICE, 2006: 141–142).

8.7 Preventive interventions

It can be seen directly from the discussion in this chapter that there is a ready mechanism for preventive and health promotion strategies in relation to depression, diabetes and dementia. Wellbeing will be improved if a concerted and comprehensive strategy is developed that addresses all three conditions, which will also have an impact on CVD prevention. Figure 8.2 suggests the importance of connecting these elements together.

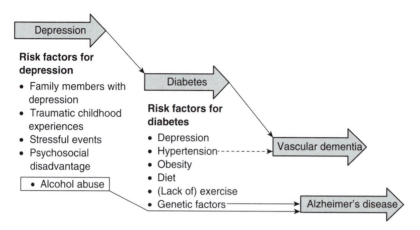

Figure 8.2   Causative pathways include depression, diabetes and dementia

From the previous discussion we know that:

- *Depression* is an important risk factor for diabetes. Risk factors for depression are shown on page 128 above and include social, psychological, familial, environmental and biological features.[16] One of the most important aspects for prevention of diabetes and wellbeing promotion is to reduce the dosage of anti-depressant medication to the minimum necessary and to apply the medication for as short a time as possible, alongside other aspects such as good self-management.
- *Type 1 diabetes* is an autoimmune disease and cannot readily be prevented, but secondary preventive strategies will focus on effective self-management.
- *Type 2 diabetes* can be prevented and a programme that focuses on the five most likely risk factors for pre-diabetes and diabetes should be put in place. The five factors are:

   o depression and its associated causative factors;
   o poor self-management, in particular not having a sensible and balanced diet;
   o obesity – excessive weight or fat deposits (adiposity) and dyslipidaemia – high cholesterol levels in the blood;
   o hypertension – high blood pressure, which may be genetically programmed or results from weight, lack of exercise and poor diet;
   o lack of exercise.

In addition to these there is evidence that over-use or abuse of alcohol has a deleterious effect on depression and diabetes. All of these factors are also associated with CVD risk.

- *Dementia* – is usually diagnosed as either vascular dementia or Alzheimer's disease. Whether Alzheimer's disease can be prevented is uncertain at the present state of knowledge, although a focus on reducing inflammation may be effective. Prevention of vascular dementia, however, flows from the discussion of depression and diabetes. Adiposity and hypertension in midlife have been shown to be risk factors for vascular dementia; diabetes has been shown to be a risk factor for LOAD.

Consequently a composite programme of identification and early treatment for depression and diabetes not only will prevent or delay the incidence of diabetes but will add to patients' overall wellbeing. In tackling the health deficits described, commissioners would be advised to fund local research on the interface of theory and practice and especially to place greater resources into geographical and human communities considered deprived in order to alleviate the prior discriminations that have left communities vulnerable. High priority interventions for diabetes and CHD include:

- school-based interventions involving meals, vending machines and policies on increased physical education;
- community-based, multi-level interventions, health education and usual care to reduce health disparities in CHD, CVD and diabetes;
- differential investment in professional support for people from deprived communities in a way that engages those communities in determining the right balance of clinical and social investment;
- alternative health care redesign strategies, such as the location of 'clinics' and other settings so as to encourage increased compliance with evidence-based guidelines and patient adherence;
- smoking cessation strategies in understudied populations such as ethnic minorities, individuals with mental illness and adolescents;
- assertive engagement with communities on traditional behavioural incentives in motivating behaviour changes (e.g. weight loss, smoking cessation, physical activity and avoiding alcohol abuse) in children and adults (Ferdinand et al., 2011).

8.8 Conclusion

Depression, diabetes and dementia are part of a continuum that starts well before the incidence of any of these diseases. It begins in the early years. Type 2 diabetes in particular can start with poor parenting and other influences such as domestic abuse that leads to low self-esteem, lack of personal care, poor nutrition, lack of exercise and obesity. Those factors are also associated with depression, and with other physical health implications such as cardiovascular disease. Many people, however, do not have unhappy and violent childhoods but still suffer the effects of diabetes and depression, and may go on to have dementia. This points to more emphasis on self-care, self-esteem, weight management, good nutrition and healthy lifestyles as well as adequate exercise through health promotion at an individual level as well as at a social level. Stopping smoking and reducing alcohol intake are both important additional features of a preventive strategy. The role of preventive services and mental health promotion will, in the long run, not only save lives but a lot of money as well.

Notes

1 High blood sugar, in which an excessive amount of glucose circulates in the blood, often as a result of diabetes mellitus. Hyperglycaemia is usually caused by low insulin levels (Type 1 diabetes) and/ or by cellular resistance to insulin (Type 2 diabetes). A person with a consistent range between c.5.5 mmol/l and 7 mmol/l is considered hyperglycaemic, whilst above 7 mmol/l is generally held to have diabetes. Chronic levels exceeding 7 mmol/l (125 mg/dl) can produce organ damage.

2   Diabetic nephropathy is a progressive disease caused by diseased blood vessels in the kidney due to longstanding diabetes mellitus, and is a prime indication for dialysis in the UK and other Western countries. It can be seen in patients with chronic diabetes and after about five years in Type 1 diabetes. Clinical nephropathy is the leading cause of premature death in young diabetic patients. Diabetic nephropathy is the most common cause of chronic kidney failure and end-stage kidney disease in the United States, http://en.wikipedia.org/wiki/Diabetic_nephropathy (accessed 28 April 2012).

3   Retinopathy is a manifestation in the eye of systemic disease; diabetes is the leading cause of new cases of blindness in those aged 20–74, with other visual manifestations such as diabetic retinopathy and macular oedema affecting up to 80% of those who have had the disease for 15 years or more, http://en.wikipedia.org/wiki/Ocular_manifestation_of_systemic_disease. (accessed 28 April 2012).

4   Narrowing or disease of the tiny blood vessels in the brain potentially leading to stroke or transient ischaemic attacks (TIAs).

5   Diabetic neuropathies are a family of nerve disorders caused by diabetes. Some people may have symptoms such as pain, tingling or numbness (loss of feeling) in the hands, arms, feet and legs, and can occur in every organ system. Between 60% and 70% of people with diabetes have some form of neuropathy. Diabetic neuropathies also appear to be more common in people who have problems controlling their blood glucose, as well as those with high levels of blood fat and blood pressure and those who are overweight.

6   Type 1 diabetes (T1DM) is a form of diabetes that results from autoimmune destruction of insulin-producing beta cells of the pancreas and leads to increased blood and urine glucose. Incidence varies from 8 to 17 per 100,000 in Northern Europe and the US, with a high of about 35 per 100,000 in Scandinavia, to a low of one per 100,000 in Japan and China (Kasper et al., 2005). It is worth noting that the incidence of MS, also an autoimmune disease, is higher in Scandinavia too. We shall consider this aspect when we look at the genetic aspects of diabetes.

7   UK Prospective Diabetes Study Group, 1998, quoted inAACE Diabetes Care Plan Guidelines (2011).

8   www.nice.org.uk/aboutnice/qualitystandards/qualitystandards.jsp (accessed 15 January 2013).

9   MSD is the UK subsidiary of Merck & Co., Inc and develops diabetes-related products.

10   Primary and secondary prevention of diabetes columns extracted from Narayan et al. (2012).

11   Primary and secondary prevention of depression columns extracted from NICE (2009a).

12   NICE (2009b).

13   Medication must be carefully prescribed as there is some evidence psychoactive medication may make diabetes worse. Opportunistic screening in primary care for sub-threshold depression in combination with minimal contact psychotherapy may be cost effective (80% likelihood) (van den Berg et al., 2007).

14   Interactome: defined as a set of molecular interactions in cells as a biological network, and includes physical interactions amongst molecules and indirect genetic interactions.

15   www.netdoctor.co.uk/diseases/depression/depressionandphysicalillness_000601.htm (accessed 19 November 2012).

16   Having given birth recently (PPD) as a risk factor is covered in Chapter 7 on children and families and is not only a risk factor for the woman but also a lifetime risk for the baby/child of lower intellectual and social functioning as well as specific disorders such as depression.

CHAPTER 9

Social Relationships and Health: Mental Wellbeing for People at Risk of Social Isolation

Social relationships – connecting with other people and playing a role in the local community – are consistently identified by the research as critical to positive wellbeing. As we noted in Chapter 2, collectivist conceptions of mental wellbeing stress the interdependence of personal wellbeing on that of familial wellbeing and social belonging. In this chapter we consider this in relation to two groups at significant risk of social exclusion – people with a mental illness and older people.

9.1 Introduction

Up to this point we have taken a broadly life course approach to health and wellbeing, but here we will consider wellbeing for those people who we might refer to as socially isolated or having particular 'vulnerabilities'. This is not the most comfortable of phrases but is intended to address the needs of people with a range of disabilities and specific needs such as people with learning disabilities or mental illness, frail elderly people (other than those with dementia – see Chapter 8), and a range of other problems that are all amenable to wellbeing interventions that will improve the quality of life and contain a preventive element, thus reducing the likelihood of pressure on services. We will deal first with mental illness and second with the needs of older people in the wider community. The common factors are the importance of wellbeing and the types of interventions that are available.

9.2 Mental health and illness

There is good evidence that long-term disability is associated with moderate to large drops in happiness or hedonic wellbeing (effect sizes ranged from 0.40 to 1.27 standard deviations), but more importantly there was (in a study by Lucas, 2007) little adaptation over time. Adaptation as a process (in this case of hedonic effects, or fairly straightforward 'happiness' rather than the more general 'flourishing') is the route that individuals take in returning to starting levels of happiness following a change in life circumstances. Lucas concluded that long-term disability is associated with long-term lasting changes in subjective wellbeing (Lucas, 2007). One of the problems of measuring wellbeing changes is adaptation effects. Some people adapt quite well to disease or disability and do not complain or consider themselves as badly off as a (non-affected) person might think they would be given the level of change in their lives (see, for example, the discussion in Heginbotham, 2012: Chapter 7). Conversely, in another study, adolescents with learning disabilities had twice the risk of emotional distress, and females were at twice the risk of attempting suicide than their peers. Yet, whilst the authors noted that educational achievement of those with a learning disability was below that of their peers, the degree of 'connectedness' to school was comparable (as was connectedness to parents). Connectedness was identified most strongly with diminished emotional distress, suicide attempts and violence (Svetaz et al., 2000).

One of the most significant topics discussed briefly in Chapters 1 and 2 is the importance of distinguishing positive mental health and wellbeing from mental illness. Mental health might be considered the 'full spectrum of mental health states' (Weich et al., 2011: 23) but in practice is frequently used to mean mental illness or mental health services. Where we differ from Weich and colleagues is in considering mental illness and mental wellbeing to be two separate, albeit related, independent continua. We use the term mental illness to mean those conditions that have been diagnosed or treated, although that terminology medicalises mental distress (and is a terminology we are keen to refute); and we use mental wellbeing to mean that continuum which refers to positive (mental) health and wellbeing. There cannot be only one spectrum that stretches from mental illness at one end to mental wellbeing at the other. Indeed Weich and colleagues make this point themselves in their paper when they suggest that people with mental illnesses can simultaneously experience mental wellbeing (Weich et al., 2011: Abstract). In a similar way to the two axes of the DSM IV diagnostic schema, a two continua model places mental illness and mental health as related but distinct dimensions (Westerhof and Keyes, 2010).

In what is a conceptually clever paper (not withstanding our disagreement about terminology and definition), Weich et al. (2011) demonstrate two significant points: first, that mental wellbeing itself has two dimensions, the hedonic and the eudaimonic, that overlap but are independent; and second, that individuals with a common mental disorder can also experience mental wellbeing. For both hedonic and eudaimonic wellbeing scores, individuals without common mental disorders demonstrate a positive slope on the graph with a strong correlation between percentage of responders and either hedonic or eudaimonic score. The slopes are slightly different but are both positive. Those with concomitant mental illness, however, show a different pattern. Again the curves are different but both demonstrate a curve that peaks at 4 (for the hedonic scores) or between 5 and 6 (for the eudaimonic scores) before dropping off towards higher scores. The hedonic trace is higher at almost 18% of respondents, whereas the eudaimonic score peaks at around 15%.

If we compare the eight factors recommended by Health Scotland (Parkinson, 2007) and quoted in 'Improving mental wellbeing in Oxfordshire' (Burton and Hitch, 2012) with the factors used by Weich et al. (2011), we can see that the two schemes used correlate fairly well with the exception of two from the nine used by Weich et al. Their scheme gives greater weight to hedonic than eudaimonic concepts of wellbeing, and less weight to emotional intelligence, the one value that does not have a corresponding

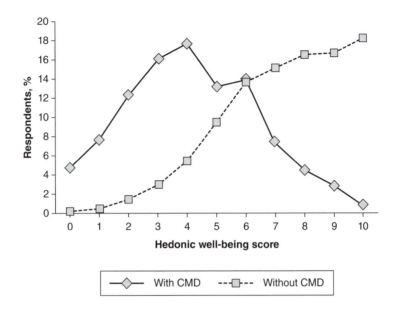

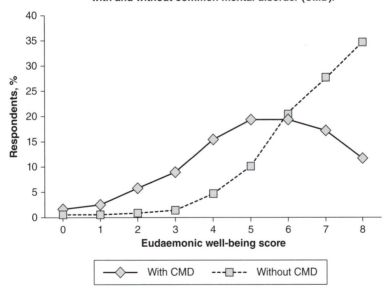

Figure 9.1 Graphs of hedonic and eudaimonic wellbeing (reproduced by permission of the Royal College of Psychiatrists)

factor in the Weich et al. scheme. This does not suggest that Weich et al.'s scheme is wrong, or that the list in the Oxfordshire paper (Burton and Hitch, 2012) is better. Rather, it offers a warning that differing analyses lead to differing conceptions of wellbeing; giving hedonic wellbeing greater weight implicitly advises that many people are interested mainly in personal happiness than in the wider flourishing of their family community.

This discussion also recommends the need for a common set of factors that will enable better understanding of differences between cohorts over time, and will enable greater clarity about the interventions that may be valuable. If we place a greater weight on hedonic wellbeing we may be tempted to invest in those interventions that appear to improve personal happiness instead of achieving a better balance of hedonic and eudaimonic outcomes that are socially more beneficial. Designing interventions to improve optimism, relationships with family members, task completion and a sense of belonging may be a little more difficult to achieve but will be ultimately more rewarding. Of course, the pursuit of happiness is an important objective for many people. However, unexpectedly little systematic research has focused on ways of increasing and sustaining happiness, 'probably because of pessimism engendered by the concepts of genetic determinism and hedonic adaptation' (Lyubomirsky et al., 2005: 112). Lyubomirsky et al. suggest that 'happiness-relevant activities and practices' offer the best way to achieve sustainable wellbeing.

Wellbeing interventions available fall into three broad categories: those that support strategies to improve belonging within the community or to a social group; those that encourage improvements in family dynamics or tackle destructive family and intimate personal relationships; and those that encourage emotional intelligence in dealing with personal problems. For example, there is evidence that, whilst people with higher levels of depressive symptoms have social lives that are less 'desirable' than those of others, those with higher level symptoms respond more strongly and positively when good events occur (Steger and Kashdan, 2009). Interventions that encourage people to seek out and achieve positive social interactions are likely to realise higher levels of wellbeing associated with such positive interactions. Depression may sensitise people to everyday experiences of both social rejection and social acceptance and thus care is required to diminish social rejection as far as possible and encourage positive experiences of belonging. Conversely, strategies to improve 'belonging' in a social context for older people have met with success as we see below.

Ensuring good evidence-based mental health care is also an important way to encourage wellbeing amongst patients and service users in mental health care. For example, the RAID programme developed by Birmingham and Solihull Mental Health NHS Foundation Trust offers a constructive way to offer treatment and preventive support (Tadros, 2011). RAID offers a rapid response, a single point of contact and is age inclusive – it can be used with dementia patients as well as those with mental health problems or acute medical or surgical demands. It appears to offer greater satisfaction for patients, a better experience for staff and better value for money. More importantly RAID is being taken up more generally as it encourages both appropriate early intervention and appropriate earlier discharge, with improved health outcomes for the patient. A high proportion of patients in general hospitals have co-morbid mental health problems, often leading to poorer health outcomes and increased health care costs. For example, psychological problems in patients with COPD and asthma are associated with lower wellbeing, increased lengths of stay in hospital (Yellowlees et al., 1988) and increased out-patient attendance (Scharloo et al., 2000).

Evidence shows that people with severe mental illness, including depression, have a higher mortality rate in comparison to the general population, partly as a result of

Table 9.1 Comparison of two ways of measuring wellbeing

	Factor descriptions (Burton and Hitch, 2012)	Wellbeing analysis (Weich et al., 2011)[1]	Detailed question to respondents (Weich et al., 2011)[2]
Emotional wellbeing	More than the absence of psychological morbidity (e.g. anxiety and depression); a positive concept that includes happiness, vitality	h Happy	Happiness evaluation on three point scale
Life satisfaction	Overall assessment of one's life, or a comparison of a perceived discrepancy between one's aspirations and achievement; includes optimistic outlook, perception of life as pleasurable	h Full of life	Proportion of the time the person has felt full of life
Optimism and hope	Positive expectations of the future; a tendency to anticipate and plan for relatively favourable outcomes	(e) Optimistic	Likely more positive than negative experiences over the next 3–5 years
Self-esteem	A belief in one's own value, accepting personal strengths and weaknesses; sense of worth. Related to emotional safety/security; confidence in personal relationships (e.g. family)	e Getting on with family	Get on well with family and other relatives
Resilience and coping	Resistance to mental illness in the face of adversity; hardiness; earned resourcefulness; sense of coherence, i.e. confidence internal and external events are predictable; a cognitive evaluation of perceived resources to deal with perceived demands; personal control	e Complete tasks	Complete tasks at home and work

(Continued)

Table 9.1 (Continued)

	Factor descriptions (Burton and Hitch, 2012)	Wellbeing analysis (Weich et al., 2011)[1]	Detailed question to respondents (Weich et al., 2011)[2]
Spirituality	Sense of purpose/meaning in life; a sense that there is something beyond the material world; attempts to harmonise life with a deeper motivation.	h Calm and peaceful	Proportion of time recently[3] that the person has felt calm and peaceful
Social functioning	a) Good personal relationships. Quality of social networks and social cohesion; community functioning; role-related coping, social participation, social functioning, sense of belonging; valuing oneself and others; b) Social support/social networks. Interactive: emotional, instrumental or financial aid is received from one's social network; feeling esteemed.	e Belonging	Belonging
Emotional intelligence	The potential to feel, use, communicate, recognise, remember, learn from, manage and understand emotions (self and others).	h e Enjoy spare time h Lots of energy	Enjoy spare time Proportion of time that had a lot of energy

A review of scales for measuring positive mental health identified eight aspects of positive mental mental wellbeing from Burton and Hitch (2012), and nine in Weich et al. (2011), as seen in Table 9.1.

Source: Parkinson (2007), quoted in Barton and Hitch (2012) and Weich et al. (2011)

increased suicide levels but also as a result of poorer care for physical disorders such as diabetes, CVD or COPD (de Hert et al., 2009).[4] Tackling these conditions holistically will benefit patients and is likely to be cost-effective. Understanding the attitude of patients to self-management and to the reasons they develop disease in the first place will assist in offering treatments that are acceptable to patients.[5] Such an approach is consistent with recovery-based approaches that emphasise personal agency and peer support and are the hallmark of progressive service delivery.

Tackling potentially destructive relationships is both ethically important and achieves good cost-effectiveness. However, the research results are mixed. Some of the research suggests that referral to counselling or talking therapies can assist in lowering rates of intimate partner violence, although this requires both parties to agree to take part (see also Cohen et al., 2011 on the implications for children). There is also evidence that alcohol abuse ramps up the likely impact of either partner abuse (as we saw in Chapter 7) and that alcohol is implicated in serious levels of domestic abuse and postnatal depression (see, for example, Certain et al., 2008, and Armstrong and Morris, 2000). Any intervention that focuses on reducing drinking, especially by men in abusive relationships, will achieve improved mental health and cost savings for both health and social care. As the *Lancet* reported recently, even with an intervention to achieve better reporting of domestic violence to general practice the number of women referred on to appropriate agencies remained very small (Anderson et al., 2009). Nonetheless the message is clear: reducing alcohol consumption and abuse is the key to reducing domestic violence. Mechanisms to encourage men to stop or reduce drinking in a way that is culturally relevant should be commissioned actively.

One of the most interesting developments of the last ten years or so is the use of social prescribing to improve mental health and wellbeing. Social prescribing for mental health provides 'a framework for developing alternative responses to mental distress, a wider recognition of the influence of social, economic and cultural factors on mental health outcomes, and improving access to mainstream services and opportunities for people with long-term mental health problems' (Friedli et al., 2008: 3). As Friedli at al. suggest, social prescribing has the benefit of being more intelligible to most people than medical models of illness. This 'broader, holistic' approach emphasises personal experience of distress and understanding of social relationships and includes a wider recognition of the causes and consequences of mental health problems. Social prescribing enables GPs and other prescribers to offer alternatives to medical 'treatments' in ways that offer patients and service users ordinary-life opportunities that have the potential to improve their wellbeing, sometimes as the by-product of the activity prescribed.

Whilst these measures have a degree of success and are generally welcomed by service users, there is some anecdotal evidence that not all referrals from general practice are necessarily appropriate or cost-effective. Prescriptions for exercise, reading ('bibliotherapy'), participation in self-help networks or 'green gyms' may be a way to divert a person from the GP practice rather than a carefully coordinated response to the person's properly assessed need. As austerity bites, general practice (and other prescribers) will have to consider carefully the cost and cost-effectiveness of differing options. Nonetheless there is evidence that these approaches work if sensibly targeted. Social prescribing can lead to increased participation by those from the most deprived communities, thus reducing equity gradients; can reduce social exclusion and promote inclusion; can assist people actively to manage their own health (as part of a wider programme to encourage appropriate self-help behaviours); and can encourage employability (Friedli et al., 2008: 10).

9.3 Older people in the community

We now turn to the needs of older people; or rather to the opportunities and assets that older people represent. Whilst many older people may live alone and not have much money, what they have is time and experience. Time banks are a mechanism that uses hours of time rather than pounds (sterling) as a community currency: participants contribute their own skills, practical help or resources in return for services provided by fellow time bank members. One of the first UK time banks was established at the Rushey Green Group Practice medical centre in 1999 and now has 200 individual members who, for example, undertake befriending and check up on patients discharged from hospital (nef, 2002; Rushey Green Time Bank, 2009; Knapp et al., 2010). Time banks are appreciated by people locally and appear to be a valued form of voluntary contribution. Most of the organisation is also done by volunteers and is inherent in the structure. Care needs to be taken with the type of activities offered but, by and large, Knapp and colleagues (2010) found that the value of the 'gift' was three times the cost of provision. Time banks have been suggested as particularly helpful in providing for older people where it is possible for retirees to offer support to working families (in the shape of baby sitting and so on) in return for gardening or minor house repairs.

As we saw in Chapter 2, one meta-analysis of information available from 63 countries (covering over 400,000 persons) demonstrated that 'individualism' was a consistently better predictor of subjective wellbeing than money, after controlling for variations in measurement technique, sample size and the time when the differing studies were undertaken. Despite some fairly obvious interactions between 'wealth' and individualism, the overall results suggest that greater personal autonomy is consistently associated with more wellbeing (Fischer and Boer, 2011). There is evidence that when one group (say Mexican-Americans) rates another (such as Anglo-Americans), they will give stronger ratings the wealthier they (the raters) are (Chana et al., 2011). This somewhat counterfactual (and possibly rather too American!) effect may have implications for research on wellbeing *if* we find that moderately high status researchers make incorrect judgements of wellbeing for those whom they are rating.

Wealth may influence wellbeing via its ability to enable persons to have more choices; but it does not reduce anxiety, and this is an especially important finding in relation to the elderly. Often older people have little wealth but a lot of time, and subjective wellbeing derives from being able to use their autonomy to good effect. Commissioners therefore can improve wellbeing by finding interventions that heighten autonomy and control without necessarily spending large sums of money. Social prescribing of time banks, walking or exercise groups, encouraging isolated older people to offer to baby sit, and similar activities, all improve wellbeing and general functioning. Many older people, the so-called 'silver surfers', now 'need less help from social services, have sorted their bills on-line, made friends with their grandchildren via Facebook and have ceased to be housebound, powerless and passive' (Turner, 2012). This is perhaps too simplistic but does demonstrate that for some older people at least, the internet is liberating. We need to seek those same outcomes for all older people.

A sense of belonging and social inclusion for older people will improve wellbeing, reduce isolation and loneliness and lower cost. One of the lower cost options is to improve exercise and give older people the chance to engage in group walking or aerobics. Whether the positive results are due to the exercise itself or due to exercising in a group of broadly like-minded individuals is a moot point. Nonetheless, exercise, physical activity and physical activity interventions have beneficial effects over several physical and mental health outcomes, including physical disorders such as obesity, cancer, cardiovascular disease and sexual dysfunction. Furthermore, there is evidence that physical activity reduces the impact of depression and improves mood (Penedo and Dahn, 2005) and that targeting of at-risk groups (e.g. older people discharged from hospital) potentially offers better returns on an investment in befriending (Knapp et al., 2011).

Older people value 'that little bit of help' to enable them to retain autonomy, choice, control and dignity in their lives, but it has become increasingly difficult to secure (Innes et al., 2006). Hours available from social services are declining for many clients although those with high levels of need have retained support. The Joseph Rowntree Foundation (2005) costed a 'Baker's Dozen' interventions ranging from help at home, through primary night care and the Cinnamon Trust programme of pet care, to befriending services or assisting school children to grow vegetables, all ranked by older people to reflect their priorities. As Rowntree (2005) suggest, some of these approaches were innovative, many were valued, everyday solutions; some were rooted in health or social care, others in the wider needs of older people. All were what we might describe as relatively cheap examples of interventions that encourage independence and reduce pressure on state services.[6] Interestingly 'community mentoring' for older people was not found to confer any benefits (Dickens et al., 2011). One study in the USA looked at the role nursing plays in supporting patients and in encouraging wellbeing. They found the need 'to change the focus of care from reactive management to a proactive prevention orientation to improve the wellbeing of older people' (Suhonen et al., 2011: 883); the results 'provide a more positive view about the state of individualized care than earlier studies' and would mean challenging the role of nurse professionals and developing a new model for older people's care (Suhonen et al., 2011: 893).

A review paper from the USA (by Yen et al., 2009) found that little research had been done on the extent to which neighbourhoods affected an older person's health. Overall they were able to say that they did, but were a little vague on the reasons. Of all the demographic variables they considered there were six that emerged as especially important: socio-economic composition, racial composition, demographics, perceived resources and/or problems, physical environment and social environment. Another study (Deeg and Thomese, 2005) showed that low-income older adults who lived in high-status neighbourhoods had poorer physical functioning, worse self-rated health, poorer cognitive ability and were lonelier than low-income adults who lived in low-status neighbourhoods (this somewhat counter-intuitive conclusion has been found in other similar studies suggesting that neighbourhoods influence health in complex ways).

Another study in the UK found little correlation between community deprivation and mental wellbeing amongst older people, although those with a sense of community cohesion had higher levels of wellbeing (measured on the Warwick Edinburgh Mental Wellbeing Scale – WEMWBS), which was not influenced by social class, income, presence of limiting long standing illness, disability or mobility problems or perceived support. This is surprising but suggests the need to repeat the study, perhaps with a different measurement scale. As the authors indicate, the way older people feel about their neighbours and neighbourhood may be important for positive mental wellbeing in later life (Gale et al., 2011). For people living in deprived areas in Glasgow, it was not only the quality of housing and the way the neighbourhood appeared (how pleasing it was to look at), but other factors were as important: 'feelings of respect, status and progress that may be derived from how places are created, serviced and talked about by those who live there' (Bond et al., 2012: 48). The implication for regeneration activities is that engaging with people in communities is as important for wellbeing as the physical structure of the neighbourhood, in particular the housing provided. However, this does not go so far as to include 'community mentoring' of older people as we saw above (Dickens et al., 2011).

Crime and the fear of crime affects the way people perceive their neighbourhood. In a paper on the theoretical links between crime, fear of crime, the environment and wellbeing, Lorenc et al. (2012: 757 (see also p.762)) suggest that crime and the fear of crime have substantial implications for wellbeing, but that the causal 'pathways are … indirect, mediated by environmental factors, difficult to disentangle and not always in the expected direction'. The built environment has multiple effects and the causal links are unclear. Nonetheless, as Lorenc and colleagues show, indirect effects of neighbourhood crime are associated with all-cause mortality (Wilkinson et al., 1998), CHD (Sundquist et al., 2006), preterm and low birth weight (Messer et al., 2006), poorer psychological health (Fowler et al., 2009) and victimisation. Many avoidance measures may themselves undermine social contacts, which may make people more anxious, and this may exacerbate poor mental health problems for those who may be more likely to suffer violence. As we can see from Figure 9.2, concerns about crime affect all aspects of the theoretical model.

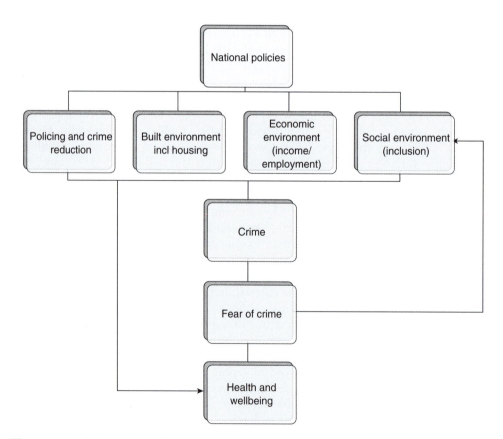

Figure 9.2 A theoretical diagram of the way that fear of crime feed into all aspects of the model (based on the text of Lorenc et al. (2012), and redrawn by the authors)

Burton et al. (2011) demonstrated a number of factors that ought to be considered in deciding the places of care for older people. Their research focused on the factors that make an area more or less safe and satisfying as a place to live: greenery, density, location, street pattern, block size, street topography and 'setback' (of dwellings from the street). Unsurprisingly older people rate safety highly, especially from traffic and crime. The research suggests that wellbeing is enhanced by recognising these fears. A potentially difficult balance needs to be struck between neighbourhoods that are safe yet encourage and maximise autonomy. As Mottusa and colleagues (2012) explain, the neighbourhood in which older people live plays a crucial role in how satisfied older people are with various aspects of their life.

One factor relevant to mental wellbeing is the impact of deprivation. Bellis et al. (2012) found that financial deprivation was strongly related to poorer wellbeing with a two-fold difference between the most and the least deprived (see also the discussion on health equity in Chapter 3). Better self-assessed health status, being retired or in a relationship were protective against low mental wellbeing. Unemployment increased the risk that those in the most deprived group would suffer low mental wellbeing, although South Asian ethnicity (perhaps because of extended family networks, cultural and religious ties) and higher levels of exercise were protective (Bellis et al., 2012; Kennedy et al., 1998).

Another example of supporting older people is a 'lifestyle-oriented occupational therapy intervention', which has been shown to have beneficial effects for ethnically diverse older people recruited from a wide array of community settings (Clark et al., 2012). Intervention participants, compared to untreated controls, showed statistically significant improvements for such things as vitality, social functioning, mental health, life satisfaction and depressive symptomatology. The intervention group had a significantly greater increase in quality-adjusted life: the cost for one QALY was around £25,000, which is less than the NICE threshold of £30,000. Because it is cost-effective and can be implemented on a broad basis, it has the potential to help reduce health decline and promote wellbeing in older people.

One important aspect of enhancing social functioning and mental health is in reducing the likelihood of suicide or self-harm amongst elderly people. Although suicide remains an uncommon event amongst older people in the UK, suicide rates do increase with age, mainly as a result of eminently treatable depression, especially amongst older men. One systemic intervention that could assist in reducing suicide still further is to improve the involvement and availability of professional social work. Most care for older people with mental health problems is provided by medical, nursing and psychological staff but the availability of social work staff as part of the team could, 'use social work skills in opening channels of communication between other professionals; communicating with carers; advocating on behalf of individuals with mental health problems; and offering acceptable and accessible support' (Manthorpe and Illife, 2011: 131). This article suggests that more emphasis should be on guideline development and on engaging social work staff in supporting older people directly by tackling sub-optimal care and support.

What does this discussion show about mental wellbeing and the role of CCGs and HWBs in commissioning and their influence on social networks, opportunities and resources? Perhaps the most salient aspect is the quality of neighbourhoods. On this analysis, HWBs can do no better than a careful assessment of the neighbourhoods within the local authority's area, using the arguments of Burton and colleagues (2011) to improve safety and promote social cohesion. Of course, no local authority can quickly or easily change the environment or undertake the sort of social engineering implied in

Burton et al.'s results. But safety, greenery and cohesion should inform any detailed strategic plan for older people. Many of the proposals on social prescribing from a few years ago – such as enhancing green spaces – will improve wellbeing more generally. Opportunities for exercise are important, and if this is in a group it can break down isolation without that being necessarily the stated objective; it is the quality of relationship and the perceptions of safety that appear to be paramount in older people's minds.

9.4 Conclusion

A great deal has been written about mental health promotion and prevention and we did not want to duplicate that here. In this chapter we have sought to identify two broad strands of health promotion and prevention: first, the importance of recognising that mental health promotion and the prevention of mental illness are two largely quite different topics although they are linked through the importance of providing positive mental health for people with mental disorders; and second, the need to consider the environment in offering wellbeing interventions to older people. So often this is brought down to considerations of green space and 'walking and talking' therapies – in other words, staying healthy through communal group exercise and conversation. But we must not neglect the wellbeing of those – the vast majority of us – that live in urban environments. Crime, fear of crime and the unsettling effects of living too close to people who may not share your values can be disturbing and unnerving. Wherever possible local authorities especially should consider the environment carefully in wellbeing interventions. Whilst offering alternatives to medical or other forms of costly professional care is essential (through social prescribing and similar mechanisms), most people want a safe and comfortable place to live.

Notes

1 h represents hedonic and e represents eudaimonic wellbeing.
2 All measured on a three point scale.
3 The period assessed was the preceding four weeks.
4 See, for example, the NHS West Midlands website, prepared by L. Moulin and N. Adams, at: www.westmidlands.nhs.uk/MultiProfessionalWorkforce/WorkforceSpecialists/MentalHealth/ RaidTypeServices.aspx (accessed 11 February 2013).
5 Kings College London University has undertaken considerable work on emotional attitudes to CVD, which points to ways of improving health and wellbeing through understanding patients' motivation. See the KCL website at www.kcl.ac.uk/iop/depts/psychology/research/researchareas/ healthpsych/research-areas/chronicdisease.aspx (accessed 11 February 2013).
6 The Joseph Rowntree Foundation's Older People's Inquiry itself was an example of involving older people in the shaping of policy, planning and practice and could be replicated by authorities (by CCGs and Trusts).

CHAPTER 10

Effective Implementation

The interventions and programmes considered in this book are, in general, well evidenced, but this is only part of the picture and evidence derived from local innovation and practice is important too. The focus of this chapter is considering how to extend the positive outcomes from this diverse evidence base into existing service configurations and routine practice. As this is a central concern for commissioners, this chapter builds on the discussion in Chapter 4, and therefore develops the argument that commissioning for mental wellbeing requires attention and investment not only in constituent programmes but also in the process of their implementation.

10.1 Introduction

The Oxford English Dictionary defines implementation as 'putting a plan into effect', and current thinking conceptualises implementation as a process, as well as an outcome. This process involves local actors getting to grips with the proposed programme, securing resources, changing practices and behaviours, and working with new people; so unsurprisingly, implementation will not happen all at once or proceed smoothly (Fixsen et al., 2005). As a number of authors have noted (see for example Fixsen et al., 2005; Barry and Jenkins, 2007), good ideas can be let down by poor project management and inadequate processes resulting in patchy implementation, poorly coordinated between agencies, with the programme implemented not reflecting the original intentions or design or being sustained long enough to achieve the required impact. However, there are also issues about the adaptation of the intervention to the local context and the creative agency of local stakeholders in interpreting and developing local programmes. The introduction of any programme, therefore, provides an opportunity for learning about the nature of the intervention and contribution of contextual factors to its implementation and realised outcomes, and therefore implementation has increasingly provided a focus for research.

10.2 The evidence on implementation

Current research indicates that implementation is often variable and imperfect in field settings and that the level of implementation influences outcomes. Referred to by Lee, Altschul and Mowbray (2008) as the gap between prevention science and intervention practice, it is evident that there are a broad a range of issues to consider. A central tension exists between being faithful to the programme, identified as being effective from research, and the introduction of this programme into the local context tailored to the local population (Lee et al., 2008). Ways in which this can be addressed by commissioners will be discussed in the next section, but first we briefly consider what the evidence says about implementation. The earlier chapters in this book have provided a summary of the interventions in terms of the evidence of what works. The accumulating evidence both from research and experience suggests that, although national policy might advocate this as a goal, it is no guarantee to implementation of evidence-based programmes. The view that practitioners and other local actors are passive recipients waiting for good ideas from science or government is seriously outdated and they have considerable scope in the interpretation of this evidence and in the development of promising innovations from their own practice and experience.

This section is concerned with how the evidence that we have discussed will be put into practice if the promised impact on health and wellbeing is to be realised. The two-step nature of applying evidence-based programmes has been developed by Fixsen and Blase (2005), as illustrated in Figure 10.1, who argue for both steps to be the focus for research endeavour. The central debate in translating evidence-based programmes into local contexts relates to the concept of implementation fidelity, to capture the idea that it is the quality of the implementation and the degree to which the programme is delivered as intended that is critical to replicating the success identified by research.

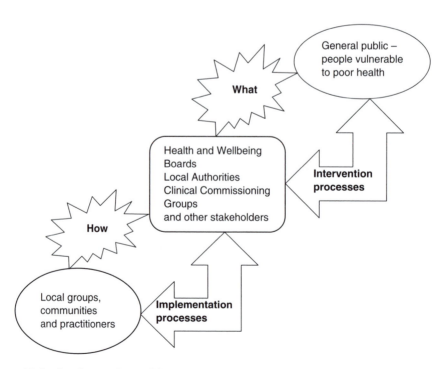

Figure 10.1   Implementing evidence-based programmes: a two-step process

Carroll et al. (2007) identified five elements of the concept of implementation fidelity from a literature review, as illustrated in Box 10.1.

Box 10.1   Aspects of implementation fidelity identified by Carroll et al. (2007)

- Adherence to an intervention: is the programme being delivered as designed?

- Exposure, dose and coverage: the amount of intervention received by the participants and whether all the people participating actually receive the intervention.

- Quality of delivery: the way in which the programme is delivered.

- Participant responsiveness: how far participants respond to or are engaged by an intervention.

- Programme differentiation: identifying which elements of the programme are essential.

Constrained by local conditions and resources, local actors may decide that doing something is preferable to doing nothing but it is evident that scant attention to the implementation process can lead to poor results and the conclusion that the evidence base is inadequate or that it does not fit the local context (Mihalic, 2002). There is a tension in the literature between those who advocate strict fidelity to the original programme and those who promote flexibility to the local context (Cross and West, 2011) and there has been a call for a greater understanding of the way in which context-level factors influence intervention uptake, success and sustainability, and the extent of context-level adaptation of an intervention or a programme (Hawe et al., 2004). Increasingly there is a recognition that implementation is a social process interwoven with the context within which it takes place (Damschroder et al., 2009). The implementation process can therefore be conceptualised as a change process both at an individual actor level and organisational level, influenced by contextual factors at a micro and macro level and by the actors involved. Therefore, planning for implementation will need to identify relevant factors at individual and organisational levels as well as the adaptability and complexity of the intervention. Critical to embedding new interventions into routine practice will be how local stakeholders engage with and make sense of the proposed changes and their workability (May, 2006). Furthermore, evidence-based practice has an implicit theory about how the programme will work (Chen, 1990) and an important aspect of the implementation process, and indeed focus for subsequent evaluation, will be articulating this theory as to how the programme will work, for who and in what contexts (Lee et al., 2008).

All of the above points to the careful planning of implementation to ensure the quality and sustainability of programme delivery and to understand the key elements of the programme and the potential for adaptation, or otherwise, in the local context. Programme development should, therefore, be based on judiciously developed underpinning theory, research principles of efficacy, and needs assessment of the target population and the settings in which the interventions will be implemented (Barry et al., 2005). Demonstrating that interventions can be implemented successfully as part of routine service delivery is an important challenge. Few interventions are sustained over time regardless of their impact, and a number of writers in this field have pointed to the importance of systems transformation to support the adoption and sustainability of evidence-based interventions. Implementing programmes in complex multi-level systems such as schools, workplaces and communities, requires a focus on the complex interaction of characteristics of the intervention, the implementer, the participants, the organisational capacity and support of the delivery system (both general and intervention-specific capacity) and the specific contexts in which the intervention is being implemented. Recognising the complexity of implementation and the importance of relevance to the local context and community are critical. The implementation components shown in Box 10.2 are essential for effective practice and an implementation checklist, derived from recommendations for implementation by Barry et al. (2005), is available in the toolkit that we developed previously (Newbigging and Heginbotham, 2010).

Box 10.2   Implementation Components for Effective Practice (Barry and Jenkins, 2007)

- Ensure readiness and commitment through active stakeholder engagement, including the participation and involvement of key intervention target groups.

- Develop a systematic planning process, building on existing practices, core principles and available evidence.

- Catalogue practical steps and practices needed for the full implementation of interventions from planning through to sustainability and service objectives.

- Identify existing supportive structures and practices across diverse sectors and services locally.

- Develop and facilitate local leadership and management for quality.

- Provide training and professional development for staff.

- Construct local organisational capacity and support including structures and resources.

- Build inter-sectoral partnerships and collaborative models with other organisations and agencies.

- Establish networks for practice knowledge exchange and transfer.

Evidence from international comparisons of implementation suggests similar lessons. We saw in Chapter 3 ways in which WHO and other international agencies have developed tools and techniques that have simple and straightforward mechanisms for undertaking equity assessments. Using those techniques judiciously alongside intervention processes described here will provide a holistic and comprehensive programme. Guidance at an international and national level is therefore important for guiding implementation at a local level including:

- publishing guidelines for effective implementation of sustainable programmes;
- setting desirable indicators by which to monitor progress;

- developing tools and designing dissemination strategies for sharing best practice;
- providing training in evidence-informed programme planning, delivery and evaluation;
- demonstrating how evidence-based practices can be mainstreamed into existing practice including detailing the supports required for effective local implementation;
- commissioning research to better understand the implementation process and the role of contextual factors on programme components.

10.3 Applying the evidence to the local context

Evidence-informed practice plays a critical role in demonstrating the success and added value of promoting public mental health and is vital to justifying funding for sustaining initiatives in the longer term. In advancing best practice locally, there is a need to focus efforts and resources on interventions and initiatives that are cost-effective, feasible and sustainable in local settings. Identification of priorities for action locally needs to be guided by strategic planning, adopting an evidence-informed approach in keeping with core principles of practice, and carried out in consultation with key stakeholders (including members of key target groups for interventions, as discussed in Chapter 4). Strategic planning should be based on findings from interventions conducted to date, systematic application of the evidence base, engagement with key stakeholders, local needs assesment, and the knowledge of practitioners and local implementers. An illustration of this from Sandwell and West Birmingham Clinical Commissioning Group is provided in Box 10.3 (NHS Confederation, 2012b).

Box 10.3   Case example: Skilling up the voluntary, community and faith sector in Tameside and Glossop to deliver wellbeing (Tameside and Glossop NHS, Tameside Strategic Partnership and Derbyshire Dales and High Peak Local Strategic Partnership (2011)

In Tameside and Glossop, to build capacity for promoting mental wellbeing at the population level, 25 mental health promotion 'champions' from statutory, voluntary and community organisations have been trained. The training, focusing on the importance of the social determinants of mental wellbeing, has enabled participants to gain greater awareness of the protective and risk factors for mental wellbeing and what needs to be, and can be, done to influence these factors.

The adoption and implementation of national and international best practice programmes within mainstream services locally, particularly the rolling out of universal progammes, will need to be considered carefully. This will include attention to available resources, both financial and human; workforce development; stakeholder engagement; and the organisational support and capacity, including leadership and interorganisational collaboration and coordination, needed to implement interventions to a high quality in the local setting. Barry and Jenkins (2007) advocate a competence enhancement approach so that the implementation process is empowering, participatory and collaborative, carried out in partnership with key stakeholders. If this is adopted the opportunities for learning about the implementation process as well as building capacity are likely to be deployed to good effect.

10.4 Building the capacity of the workforce

A skilled and trained workforce with the necessary competencies to work at population level and with groups, communities and individuals will be central to effective implementation. It is becoming increasingly clear that the resources and skills required for effective implementation tend to be underestimated, or at least not thought through sufficiently. It is also recognised that leadership is necessary at all levels, from macro policy-making through to implementation on the ground, if plans are to be realised. Whilst public mental health is indeed everybody's business, dedicated time and resources and specific competencies are needed for effective, accountable implementation. Thus, the commitment to and investment in workforce development will rest on agreements made by senior officers and reflect the priorities established and supported by HWBs and the partner organisations. Third sector and community organisations also make a major contribution to implementing best practice and therefore should also be supported to develop their workforce, as necessary.

At least two different levels of workforce may be necessary:

1 Dedicated public health and mental health promotion specialists who facilitate and support the development of policy and practice across a range of settings. These specialists bring specific expertise around interventions, their implementation and evaluation and have an important leadership and support role to play in translating plans into action on the ground.
2 The wider workforce across the different sectors – health, education, employment, community and third sector organisations – will need training in awareness raising in the value and content of health improvement activities. Some staff will need skills development to support and implement specific initiatives; health and wellbeing will also need to be a focus for continuing professional development and training to maintain the quality of practice and update the skill sets required to work within a changing context. An example of this is provided in Box 10.4

Building the capacity of the workforce in developing and implementing mental health promotion programmes is fundamental to mainstreaming and sustaining action in this area. Workforce education and training range from awareness raising and training about the promotion of mental health for the wider workforce, to skills development needed to support and implement specific initiatives, through to dedicated mental health promotion specialists who facilitate and support the development and implementation of policy and practice across a range of settings. Continuing professional development and training is required to enhance the quality of practice and update the skill set required to work within a changing context. This will require resourcing and therefore needs to form part of the strategic plan, agreed by HWBs.

10.5 Identify opportunities to mainstream interventions

It is something of a truism that effective implementation is the key to successful programmes, but one of the major barriers to effective implementation of many, if not all, health promotion programmes is their multi-factorial and multi-agency requirements. Critical to this is engaging the right partners at the most appropriate organisational level early in the process. To obtain the full benefits of most interventions it is essential to recognise the holistic nature and multi-sectoral elements of the intervention. For example, good implementation of universal and targeted support for postnatal depression needs effective coordination and team work between GPs, the primary health care team, health visitors, social workers and the mental health provider, to create a coordinated approach; interventions with elderly people may, for example, engage the voluntary sector, primary care, transport and adult education.

Central to these programmes is the role of GPs in supporting change in behavioural risk factors, promoting self-management and provision of information, working alongside care managers from social care, voluntary sector agencies and community organisations with roots in the local communities and other agencies. As GP commissioning develops, the value of social care and GPs working together to develop a proportionate universalism will be invaluable: on the one hand ensuring that messages are delivered to all without exception and simultaneously following up those where screening indicates an individual need that must be addressed.

Done well these coordinated processes enable interventions to become the mainstream offerings of a sector, in the knowledge that they are supported throughout by other agencies. One agency cannot alone sustain a programme that relies on a range of agencies for its effectiveness; but there is evidence that together a programme can generate added value through achieving a critical mass of resources focused on the population and the groups at risk.

It can be seen readily that some interventions lend themselves to becoming part of mainstream regular services: health visitor support for mothers; debt counselling; social prescribing of fitness regimes for older people. Partnership arrangements should be developed where there are well evidenced whole systems savings to be achieved as well as longer-term improvements in wellbeing. In many cases the interventions described in the ten commissioning areas include elements that may already exist or can be dovetailed into existing services. The challenge is to ensure cost-effective inclusion of these new elements in a way that is sustainable.

Demonstrating that interventions can be implemented successfully and sustained as part of routine service delivery is an important challenge. Few interventions are sustained over time regardless of their impact. It may be helpful to plan for sustainability by aligning intervention goals with local policy and service objectives, identifying existing support structures and practices, and facilitating local leadership and management for quality implementation.

Box 10.4   Case example from Sandwell and West Birmingham Clinical Commissioning Group (NHS Confederation, 2012b)

Commissioners in Sandwell (now Sandwell and West Bromwich CCG, previously Sandwell PCT) set out to respond to specific health inequalities to develop a primary care-led approach to mental health and wellbeing. A metropolitan borough, Sandwell in 2011 was the four-teenth most deprived local authority in England. Around 23% of the population comes from BME groups, mainly of South Asian heritage and the area has a number of specific chal-lenges, including high rates of unemployment and poor housing. The specific inequalities that health commissioners sought to address were:

- poor levels of mental and physical health, including low aspirations and emotional distress associated with severe deprivation at a population level;

- social deprivation;

- poor access to community mental health and wellbeing services;

- heavy use of secondary care mental health services based on a dominant psychiatric dis-ease model.

The PCT undertook a mental health GP profiling assessment and a gap analysis, identify-ing that there were high levels of mental ill-health in socially deprived wards with high unemployment and needs not being met, with a higher than average representation of BME groups in acute services but with low uptake of lifestyle services. Their assessment also high-lighted the correlations between people diagnosed with depression and other long-term conditions, particular CVD and diabetes (as noted in Chapter 8). The conclusion was the need to prioritise and make adequate provision for the treatment and prevention of depression.

The PCT appointed a primary care mental health and wellbeing lead who worked in part-nership with the Professional Executive Committee chair and mental health lead. The PCT commissioners worked with local stakeholders to develop the business case for change, building on their assessment but setting up listening events with residents and GPs to gather a detailed view of the problems and what needed to change. They also undertook asset mapping and identified which existing services could be used more effectively. The demand and the capacity of the workforce were modelled and they developed a system to collect pre- and post-outcome measures. They sourced funding and partnership opportuni-ties and actively looked for opportunities where their objectives aligned with national policy in order to secure funding.

The team developed a collaborative primary care model that combined positive self-help, psycho-education, talking therapies and access to specialist support, all developed with service users. The model is a stepped approach using different levels of intervention according to need, with the purpose of low intensity services being to empower the popu-lation to make decisions about their own care. There is a confidence and wellbeing service open to all but also targeted at those with symptoms of mild depression, obesity, medically unexplained symptoms and anxiety. This level of services includes self-help coaches and community development workers.

The approach is showing some promising early outcomes:

- 4,000 people completing prevention, wellbeing and improvement programmes, saving around £800,000 in prevention costs;

- 3,000 people have accessed talking therapies saving around £600,000.

The key learning points identified from this are:

- the continued need to align primary health care with key partners and stakeholders including probations services, schools, libraries, colleges and secondary care acute and mental health providers;

- the importance of investing in training for primary care and community care staff;

- the importance of clinical and service user engagement.

10.6 Conclusion

Explicit direction about where resources should be invested does not mean stifling local innovation; rather, creative local practice should be balanced with evidence-based programmes that have been shown to work across different settings. The adoption and implementation of national and international best practice programmes within mainstream services locally, particularly the rolling out of universal progammes, will need to be considered carefully. Adopting a best practice programme does not in itself guarantee success. It requires attention to good quality implementation, including adequate resources such as funding, staff skills, training, supervision, and the organisational support and capacity needed to implement interventions to a high quality in the local setting.

CHAPTER 11

Effectiveness and Cost-Effectiveness: Accountability for Outcomes

This chapter will make some comments on the outcomes that are achieved for the interventions described and the cost-effectiveness of those interventions. In previous chapters we have considered in some detail the interventions that have been suggested and some of the cost criteria but we have not looked at the outcomes achieved, or the cost or cost-effectiveness of those interventions. Methods of evaluating and measuring outcomes will be discussed, and with it the effectiveness of the intervention, measured against either professional or service user expectations. The thorny issue of outcomes-based commissioning will be described.

11.1 Local and national accountability for outcomes

A robust evaluation framework for local initaitives will need to be put in place in order to monitor progress in meeting desirable and measurable processes and outcomes, building up the local evidence base and collecting learning from practice. Outcomes are not simply those that professional staff have come to expect, but include the outcomes desired by service users.

Agreeing an outcomes framework for commissioning for mental wellbeing has to take account of national developments, but is also for local determination. When outcomes are being sought in relation to improving population mental wellbeing, it is important to aim for outcomes and indicators that enable comparisons across localities. Outcomes of wellbeing are more than the absence of clinical indicators of illness, and measures of positive health and wellbeing are being actively explored. For the first time work is underway at a national level to measure wellbeing: the ONS started

producing annual reports in 2012 through its Measuring National Well-being programme, and questions about subjective wellbeing have been included in the
Household Survey since 2011. The WEMWBS is also being widely used to assess
wellbeing at a local level (Tennant et al., 2007). Such measures are limited as they
focus on how people are feeling and view their life at a specific point in time, and of
course this varies. However, anecdotal evidence suggests that the instrument is valuable both for individuals and groups and reasonably reliably measures the effects of
different types of interventions.

Performance indicators should provide information about strengthening protective
factors and reducing risk factors in the social and physical environment. The new local
government Local Performance Framework should take in to account national policies
and local priorities to provide a framework that links outcome indicators with performance objectives. Work is underway to develop appropriate metrics for detecting
improvements in mental wellbeing, and quite a lot of progress has been made. Nonetheless
a lot of effort has gone into developing acceptable outcome measures (e.g. the Mental
Health Outcomes group at the Department of Health during the 1990s); what seems to
work best is some form of star diagram or spidergram that collates six or more 'dash-
board' indicators into a composite picture.

11.2 Wellbeing interventions

As we saw in Chapter 4, the process for commissioning a health and wellbeing intervention also provides the opportunity to specify in advance the outcome measures to use.
The most effective processes have some of the following elements in common. First it is
essential to decide the programme objective: is the intention to offer a universal intervention or to target specific known groups with lower health status or poor social care
outcomes. Then it will be important to decide whether the overall objective is to:

- maximise wellbeing 'gain' overall?
- target those with the lowest wellbeing?
- target those requiring additional assistance to benefit from whatever programme is offered?

In determining the population target is the intention to:

- target minority populations with specific deprivations?
- offer interventions to all members of a community or neighbourhood?
- target specific population groups, children, women, older people, etc.?
- target groups with particular conditions?

An alternative strategy is to use information from a JSNA analysis or from the preceding population targets to define programme objectives to describe outcomes and wellbeing measures. If any programme is to achieve maximum health and social gain from
the intervention then it will be necessary to identify the wider educational, social,
economic and community oriented gains to be obtained. By 'mainstreaming' interventions it will be possible to add value to existing health and social care provision wherever possible, and to develop the most cost-effective solutions whilst tackling the
agreed target group.

11.3 Evaluation of outcomes

Alongside population level data, fine-grained data, including qualitative data, is also needed to understand the meaning of mental wellbeing, the factors that influence it and potential interventions for mental health improvement across diverse communities. Furthermore, specific measures and data collection stages will need to be designed in relation to evaluating specific mental health improvement activities. The Mental Wellbeing Impact Assessment toolkit, for instance, contains examples of indicator sets that might be used or developed further for specific circumstances. Resource J (MWIA Collaborative, 2011) shows how mapping indicators to MWIA factors may suggest direct or proxy indicators. The difficulty with this approach, however, is twofold: first, measurement techniques, and second, the availability of data that is relevant in forms that make it accessible.

Let us take one example from the MWIA. Under the rubric of 'enhancing control', one of the individual factors is 'knowledge, skills and resources to make healthy choices'. The specific indicators for this one factor alone include: use of public libraries; migrants' English language skills; alcohol-harm related hospital admission rates; prevalence of Chlamydia in under 20s. Of course for a particular issue it may be sensible to use a small subset of all the possible indicators available. But most importantly it will be necessary to have indicators that are coherent for a particular factor and can be measured and collated fairly readily.

The outcome indicators that are directly relevant to health and wellbeing (DH, 2012a) are shown in Box 11.1:

Box 11.1   Outcome indicators that contain information on the wider determinants of health and health inequalities (see DH, 2012a: 11)

Indicators

- Children in poverty
- School readiness (Placeholder)
- Pupil absence
- First-time entrants to the youth justice system
- 16–18 year olds not in education, employment or training
- People with mental illness or disability in settled accommodation
- People in prison who have a mental illness or significant mental illness (Placeholder)
- Employment for those with a long-term health condition including those with a learning difficulty/disability or mental illness
- Sickness absence rate
- Killed or seriously injured casualties on England's roads

- Domestic abuse (Placeholder)

- Violent crime (including sexual violence) (Placeholder)

- Re-offending

- The percentage of the population affected by noise (Placeholder)

- Statutory homelessness

- Utilisation of green space for exercise/health reasons

- Fuel poverty

- Social contentedness (Placeholder)

- Older people's perception of community safety (Placeholder)

The list in Box 11.1 is a valuable (and comprehensive) attempt to capture information on the wellbeing aspects of health and social care in their broadest sense. However, for our purposes there are some that do not apply as much to the wellbeing agenda of prevention and health promotion. Those that do fit with the purpose of this book can be collated into four areas that match, more or less, the chapter headings of Chapters 6 to 9. For example:

- Children in poverty – reducing poverty will make a huge difference to the opportunities open to children to achieve their potential in society, and that implies also improvements in pupil absence, which may be due to domestic problems or abuse or may occur as a result of simple poverty. Measures: number of children in households below the poverty line; pupil absence statistics. (Chapter 6)
- First-time entrants to the youth justice system – linked to poor parental training and behaviours; and measures of NEETs (16–18 year olds not in education, employment or training) relate their needs to the 'life course' approach to social stress: by intervening early we can be almost certain that these numbers will reduce and young people will be able to make a positive contribution to society. Measures: number of young people designated as NEET; numbers of cautions and first offences for drug offences. (Chapter 6)
- Employment for those with a long-term health condition including those with a learning difficulty/disability or mental illness – as we saw in Chapter 7, employment remains the most important way in which people gain esteem and sufficient income for a decent life. Sickness absence rates – especially as a result of mental health problems – are important measures of the efficacy of interventions to improve employment retention and other opportunities. Measures: numbers of people with diagnosed mental disorders in employment (this will have a built in error as a result of the lack of understandable openness about mental health problems). (Chapter 7)
- Older people are especially affected by fuel poverty, and are susceptible to the availability and opportunities to utilise green space for exercise/health reasons; their perception of community safety is a factor we considered at some length in Chapter 9. Measures: surveys of older people on the benefits they enjoy from open space; surveys of older people's fear about crime and the implications of crime. (Chapter 9)

The discussion in Chapter 8 on diabetes, depression and dementia fits into the second group of service improvement suggestions described within *Improving Outcomes and*

Supporting Transparency (DH, 2012a). Our view is that there are significant preventive and health promotion aspects of the conditions and interventions described in Chapter 8, and the interventions match the life course approach that we have taken, for them to be considered here alongside the four areas shown in the bulleted list above. It is evident that intervening in those conditions (such as diabetes, but also in the other disease areas described, such as CHD) achieves preventive, health promoting and wellbeing outcomes, and is cost-effective especially in preventing disorders occurring in the first place and in ameliorating the worst aspects of disease. In other words, by intervening as early as possible (i.e. in childhood rather than waiting for disorders to appear) and comprehensively across all conditions using a person-centred approach, the impact of specific conditions can be reduced and individuals will be able to live more fulfilled lives with less disability.

The difficulty with these aspects of health and wellbeing is finding the right measures for the outcomes achieved, and being certain that they are actually measuring the outcomes of the interventions implemented (rather than simply measuring ad hoc or non-causal effects). For the four broad areas collated above we do have relevant measures, as are noted alongside each of the areas.

11.4 Effectiveness and cost-effectiveness of interventions

We describe an intervention as acceptable if it achieves the objective we have in mind; and we consider effectiveness if the intervention achieves some part or percentage of the objectives as described. But in this field, that is easier said than done, for at least three reasons. First, defining 'health' and 'wellbeing' for our purposes is anything but straightforward. In general we know what we mean, as we have shown in the previous chapters, but measuring wellbeing, as we saw above, is difficult if not impossible to do skilfully or accurately. If we cannot measure health and wellbeing readily how can we know we have made an improvement? This has bedevilled the previous chapters on specific aspects of wellbeing (Chapters 6 to 9) where we have tried to get a grip on the wellbeing outcomes.

Second, how do we know what objective to set? This partly follows from the first point: if we cannot define health or wellbeing it is difficult to establish adequately a target for improvement. But it is also because not knowing the parameters of wellbeing makes establishing a wellbeing objective problematic. For example, if we do not know the full extent of subjective wellbeing and its relation to emotional wellbeing (let alone other aspects), how can we be sure that we have the right target, or one that does not interact with another factor. As we saw in Chapter 9 there is a debate about eudaimonic and hedonic wellbeing which has not been resolved.

Third, the literature does not always tell us which component of wellbeing is the one that is affected by the intervention. Let us think for a moment about diabetes and the discussion in Chapter 8. If diabetes is a precursor for and causative of depression *in some people* but not in all, then we need to know which people and why; conversely, if depression is a precursor for and possibly *causative of* diabetes in *some* people, then again we need to understand the aetiology and causation pathways. Otherwise we may apply a universal intervention (which may of course be appropriate depending on the circumstances) to every one when only some relatively small percentage (say 20%)

have any chance of benefiting. Similarly, measuring effectiveness is problematic. Effectiveness is defined as the ratio of outcomes to inputs: do we get what we set out to achieve for a given input – such as sum of money or the work of a group of staff? Describing the input conditions has always challenged economists as it is never clear which staff, or buildings, or medicines or whatever factor is required are actually involved in this particular intervention.

The place to start is in defining what cost-effectiveness we are trying to measure. In the two-by-two matrix in Figure 11.1[1] we can see that there are two cells in which we are interested primarily, both associated with improved outcomes. First, of course, we need to ask 'improved over what?' We must have data on what works now, or what level of health or wellbeing we are achieving, before we can discuss improvements.

Decisions about what to recommend turn on what we know from research about the outcomes that have been achieved, the personnel involved and the cost of the intervention. Many of those costs are not fully assessed either for completeness (have all factors been included?) or appropriateness (have they been costed correctly and fully?) Let us consider two examples.

The first example is based on data from 20 RCTs. Knapp and colleagues concluded that mixed parenting programmes had an effectiveness rate of 33% costing on average £1,177 per family (2011 or earlier data). The outcomes were reduced use of NHS, social care and special education services and reduced crime, from age 5–30. Excluding employment costs or income, social security and adult mental health costs the return appeared to be just under £8 for every £1 spent including savings in public expenditure of just under £3. This would appear to be a good investment at a ratio of 8:1. Various parenting programmes have shown a range of returns on investment, from a cost-benefit ratio of better than 7:1 in Chicago (Reynolds et al., 2001), to approximately 10:1 offered by Sure Start (Scott et al., 2001a; Edwards et al., 2007). A cost-effectiveness analysis of parenting

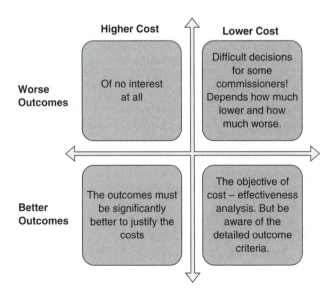

Figure 11.1 Cost-effectiveness relies on knowing how much better health and wellbeing is for the intervention suggested

programmes for parents of children at risk of developing conduct disorder found that the programme involved relatively modest costs with robust clinical outcomes, suggesting it would represent good value for public spending (Edwards et al., 2007). The costs for children who had been identified with conduct disorder at age 10, were 10 times higher than for those with no problems, and 3.5 times higher than for those with less severe conduct problems by age 28 (Scott et al., 2001a). Interventions for those with conduct disorder (some 5% of the child population) resulting in improved behaviour to the median level within the child population have been estimated as costing £210 million but saving potentially as much as £5.2 billion (Friedli and Parsonage, 2007).

Robust cost-benefit evidence is available to show that prevention and early intervention have life-time benefits over the life course and interrupt the cycle of deprivation that can occur over two or three or more generations in the same family. A number of studies have demonstrated significant cost-benefits from early years interventions (Karoly et al., 2005). 'Those most at risk will make the greatest gains from early childhood programmes and the social costs will be the highest for a failure to intervene on their behalf' (Campion, 2009). However, whilst there *is* good evidence of cost-effectiveness, not all interventions work as well as the best, and some prevention and early intervention programmes fail to generate more benefits than costs (Aos et al., 2004). A cost-benefit analysis was conducted by Karoly et al. (2005) for home-visiting programmes serving at-risk children and for early childhood education progammes serving low-income three and four year olds. For five of the seven studies the estimates of the net benefits per child served range from about $1,400 per child to nearly $240,000 per child. Even the most expensive programmes have been found to pay for themselves by the time the children are four years old (Olds, 2002).

A second example is of a health promotion programme undertaken through the place of employment. The intervention was a 'multi-component health promotion programme including health risk appraisal and information … tailored to the employees' readiness to change health related behaviours' (Knapp and McCrone, 2011). Whilst the intervention cost only £80 per annum per employee, the employers described reduced absenteeism, reduced stress levels and improved productivity. The main employee benefits of reduced sickness absence and less avoidable mental illness meant a saving of just under £10 for every £1 invested. Indeed, interventions to facilitate re-employment, particularly in good quality jobs, are one of the most effective ways of promoting the mental health of the unemployed (Vuori and Silvonen, 2005).

Knapp and McCrone note that the most effective of the interventions they considered were suicide prevention training courses provided to all GPs (£43.99 per £1 invested) and suicide prevention through bridge safety barriers (£54.45). However, the payback here was overwhelmingly in the private sector. Of those interventions with both public and private sector payback, the most effective by far was prevention of conduct disorder through SEL programmes (£83.73). In the middling group was early intervention in psychosis (£17.97), screening for alcohol misuse (£11.75), and school-based interventions to reduce bullying (£14.35). At the other end of the scale were a number of interventions that did not appear to be cost-effective: health visitor interventions to reduce the impact of postnatal depression (£0.80), early intervention for depression in diabetes (£0.33), or befriending for older adults (£0.44). However, we must be careful how we treat these results.

First, we should not compare lives lost with lives damaged. Suicide is absolute and does not allow for rehabilitation; other interventions concern non-final outcomes, although serious for all that. Some of the research and modelling on which the work of Knapp and colleagues (2011) is based recognises the limitations of the work. For example, the main cost of the health visitor interventions to reduce the impact of postnatal depression is training for health visitors (£1400), which is difficult to recoup in one year. The authors of that section of the report (Annette Bauer, Martin Knapp, David McDaid) agree that the results are conservative and that lower treatment costs and a reduced productivity loss are outweighed by increased training and higher staff costs for providing the interventions. As they go on to say, however, 'if it is assumed that depressive symptoms persist after one year, it is likely that cost savings could be achieved in the medium term as treatment costs and productivity loss would be further reduced. Longer term, it would be important to include in any evaluation the economic costs of negative behavioural, emotional and cognitive consequences for the children of mothers who suffered from postnatal depression' (Knapp et al., 2011: 4). In other words, whilst at first blush the intervention does not appear to be cost-effective, over a longer time frame in which a child might be prone to behavioural problems this becomes a potentially valuable intervention. Overall the results show a significant improvement in the quality of life for mothers and the cost-effectiveness of the intervention is similar to the findings of Morrell et al. (2009).

Similarly, the figures for diabetes and depression are rather misleading. The report by Derek King, Iris Molosankwe and David McDaid (within Knapp et al., 2011: 31) is based on a collaborative care model which can be delivered in a primary care setting to individuals with co-morbid diabetes and depression. Collaborative care includes GP advice and care, the use of antidepressants and CBT for some patients. The difference with usual care is that a GP practice nurse acts as a case manager for patients receiving care; GPs also incur additional time costs liaising with practice nurses. One of the first things to note about this is that it is based heavily on the pathology of the disorder and does not encompass an assets-based approach. The treatment pathway is GP-primary care managed rather than community managed. Second, with an alternative lifestyle improvement programme run by a mental health provider and possibly a social enterprise, it is likely an improvement would be made in both costs and outcomes. The estimated benefits do not include productivity losses due to premature mortality, further quality of life gains associated with avoidance of the complications of diabetes, such as amputations (cost from £8,500), heart disease (non-fatal myocardial infarction £4,000), renal failure or other complications. Nor does the analysis include long-term cost savings from reduced complications. But most importantly, assessing patients for both depression and diabetes will identify those for whom self-care is a problem and where lifestyle risk factors predominate.

One area that is of significant concern to the government, the health service, social care and to local authorities generally is abuse and misuse of alcohol. As the UK government's actions in late 2012 and early 2013 suggest, the most cost-effective approach in high income/consumption countries such as the UK is to set a minimum price per unit of alcohol, mainly because it affects all alcohol consumers and has a broad population impact in reducing morbidity (Chisholm et al., 2004). Early interventions in hazardous drinking are both effective and cost-effective (Chisholm et al., 2004). NICE (2007) estimates of the cost per QALY gained by screening and brief interventions range from £1,500 to £11,800, well below the NICE cost-effectiveness threshold of approximately £30,000, and all of the estimates cited in the report disregard a series of additional benefits, such as benefits to other family members of those who misuse alcohol, lower crime costs, less intimate partner violence, higher employment and improved productivity. Campion (2009) reports that an estimated 30% of

A&E visits per annum are related to alcohol; 70% of weekend A&E attendances between midnight and 5am may be alcohol related (Drummond et al., 2003); one in every 15 A&E visits goes on to become a hospital admission; one nurse could avert around 40 admissions per annum at a saving to the NHS of approximately £45,000.

Table 4.1 demonstrates the ten most sensible investment areas and indicates the range of investments that can be made which will have a reasonably good chance of being cost-effective. For example, Commissioning Area 1 (Good parental health) shows a return after one or two years on even the most expensive programmes. Area 2 (parenting skills) is highly cost-effective with significant savings to the public purse. These programmes achieve a relatively quick return on investment, with costs for children with conduct disorders, for example, reducing to a fifth after only 18 months. Similarly, building social and emotional resilience of children using an integrated approach with universal and targeted interventions in primary schools is highly effective. The cost-effectiveness of these interventions is clear, but using methods to calculate the social return on investment (SROI), the value for other interventions may also become more readily apparent. SROI is increasingly being used by commissioners and other organisations to understand the social and environmental, as well as the economic, benefits that are being created (Goodspeed et al., 2009). This approach fits well with a values-based approach to commissioning.

11.5 Conclusion

The evidence given here provides powerful proof that prevention and health promotion – focusing on health and wellbeing (with a distinct flavour of positive mental health) – is both cost-effective and socially worthwhile. Many of the interventions cited show extensive benefits at moderate cost; in some cases there is a ten-fold cost improvement over doing nothing. Of course, it is not true of everything, and for some interventions we have only very rough estimates of cost *or* benefit. However, there is no doubt that early childhood and school interventions are highly cost-effective, workplace support can save significant sums and interventions to tackle alcohol abuse and misuse should be commissioned by every health and social care commissioner in the UK. Long-term conditions (diabetes, COPD and neurological disorders) will benefit from focused wellbeing interventions, notably but not only to improve self-management of the condition. Finally, the importance of health and wellbeing for older people and for people living with long-term mental disorders must be emphasised.

Note

1 Based on Professor Martin Knapp (PSSRU, London School of Economics) and Professor Paul McCrone (King's College London, Institute of Psychiatry), speaking at a conference on Best Practice in Mental Health GP Led Commissioning, 25 March 2011. See also Knapp et al. (2011).

CHAPTER 12

Preventive and Health Promoting Strategies

12.1 Introduction

This final chapter is short and to the point! Our interest here is to encourage senior NHS and social care managers, as well as those in third sector organisations, to take the proposals in this book seriously. The Quality, Innovation and Productivity (QUIP) programme (to which another P for Prevention was later added) within the NHS offers the opportunity to transform the way professional staff work, by developing holistic personalised care that recognises the interplay of differing elements of disease profiles and preventive agendas. For example, we have made the point strongly within the text that depression, diabetes and dementia should be considered together wherever possible. Similarly, we believe that alcohol consumption demands a major assertive programme to change personal behaviours, which could become cost-effective rapidly. We need a life course approach to many other disorders: for instance, if children are not supported correctly in their early years they are likely to go on to have poorer educational attainment, to look after themselves less well than others and thus to develop a range of physical and mental health problems earlier.

Although a large part of this book has been about health and wellbeing from a positive mental health perspective, many of the arguments apply to the *anti-wellbeing* effects of physical diseases and disorders. Promoting positive mental health for all is essential; but so is tackling those disorders that reduce overall wellbeing. It seems to us perverse that we might promote social prescribing of walking groups only to ignore the major implications for wellbeing of CVD, diabetes, COPD and other chronic disorders.

12.2 Acceptance of the value of preventive and health promoting strategies

We hope that senior NHS and social care managers will recognise the savings that will accrue over a relatively short timeframe from implementing the various interventions described here. In particular, it is essential to consider the veracity of claims for economic impact. Some interventions have payback periods of a year or so, others rather longer. But importantly all offer health improvements that are cost-effective. We understand that many senior managers remain to be convinced of the economic arguments in the current financial context and their concerns about additional likely cuts to social care especially. And yet we hear more prejudice than reason in managers' assessments of preventive and promoting interventions, often on an untested assumption that 'prevention takes a long time'. Sometimes it does, sometimes it doesn't; but if we don't start sometime, it never will!

All NHS and local authority social care organisations, as well as most private and independent providers, want the best results and outcomes for the money they invest. That seems uncontentious. In order to achieve this, however, requires an acceptance, not slavishly but intelligently, of the cost and outcomes of doing things differently. If we do not focus on a positive assets-based public health we will continue to attack evident pathology without mobilising community assets to our advantage; without recognising the huge problems that poor care in the early years creates, we will continue to pay over many years for poor self-care in a host of chronic diseases. There is a cumulative impact across the whole system. This thus begs a question: how do we measure the impact of these interventions? We will need improved metrics for capturing the effects of change and we need to be honest about the outcomes we achieve. The UK government has made a start, although many of these so-called outcome measures are really process measures.[1] The NHS Outcomes Framework is based on five domains concerned to achieve high-level national outcomes that the NHS should be aiming to improve. It focuses on:

- Domain 1 Preventing people from dying prematurely;
- Domain 2 Enhancing quality of life for people with long-term conditions;
- Domain 3 Helping people to recover from episodes of ill health or following injury;
- Domain 4 Ensuring that people have a positive experience of care; and
- Domain 5 Treating and caring for people in a safe environment; and protecting them from avoidable harm. (DH, 2011a)

Domain 2 is the appropriate place to include wellbeing outcome targets, and it is possible that this will form a component of the Department of Health's work over the coming two years or so.

The government insists that it wants health care outcomes, public health outcomes and adult social care outcomes to be the best in the world. To achieve this the Department of Health is developing three strategic outcomes frameworks – the NHS Outcomes Framework, the Public Health Outcomes Framework and the Adult Social Care Outcomes Framework. Although the three outcomes frameworks are intended to bring focus, there are many who believe that aligning the outcomes across the frameworks and setting shared national level outcomes, with shared accountability, will lead to improved implementation. The Public Health Outcomes Framework for England, 2013–2016 (DH, 2012a), sets out a series of outcome indicators based on achieving an overarching vision for public health under four domains:

- Improving the wider determinants of health with indicators related to tracking progress in factors that affect health and wellbeing;
- Health protection with indicators related to protecting population health form wider threats;
- Health improvement with indicators related to enabling people to make healthy choices and including self-reported measures of wellbeing;
- Healthcare and premature mortality with indicators relating to mortality.

These indicators may assist in understanding progress on improving and protecting health. The Social Care Outcomes Framework also has four outcome domains, two of which also provide a home for wellbeing targets, namely:

- Enhancing quality of life for people with care and support needs; and
- Delaying and reducing the need for care and support.

Unhappily the extent of the reorganisation at the time of writing is likely to delay any reasonable grip on the agenda for at least one year and probably two, at a time when resource shortages are biting. We hope that health and social care managers will implement this agenda as soon as possible.

Mental health care has, as WHO describes, a 'vicious cycle of mental disorder and social disadvantage (Blas and Kurup, 2010: 118). Within this 'vicious cycle' is a self-reinforcing loop that builds on poor educational attainment, imposing stressful life events as well as alcohol abuse and substance use, with the implications of discrimination on the grounds of gender and ethnicity discrimination. These factors lead to higher probability of the need for mental health services, which in turn fuels social exclusion. Social exclusion feeds stressful life events and the cycle continues. Once this has started it is difficult to stop without a very concerted effort. Although we have argued throughout that positive mental health is for everyone, we must challenge those who do not understand the importance of changing the way society operates, such that people with mental illnesses are treated as we would treat anyone else, and so that resources are diverted to the best possible care and support that money can buy, and the highest wellbeing available.

Evidence exists of significant activity but a lack of strategic coordination. Leadership and accountability are in short supply. It is not (usually) a problem of capacity but rather of 'faith' based on good hard evidence. Martin Knapp and colleagues (Knapp et al., 2011) have shown that many of the mental health interventions are cost-effective, albeit in some cases marginally. By implementing the interventions described it should be possible to get both the benefits of prevention and the expectations of health promotion. Mental health is an essential component of general health (RCPsych, 2010; DH, 2011); mental wellbeing is more than absence of mental illness. Mental wellbeing is a key social asset of economic significance as a resource for long-term social and economic prosperity. Wellbeing is the other side of the coin of personalisation – an opportunity for greater personal responsibility in health and social care. Mental wellbeing and physical illness are connected with long-term health conditions, particularly CHD, CVD, hypertension, diabetes and obesity, and thus addressing mental wellbeing is key to local action to tackle health inequalities.

Responsibility for promoting mental wellbeing extends across all disciplines and government departments. Despite our reservations expressed in Chapter 1, it will be important to position much of the guidance in the mental health policy world at the interface with proposals on recovery, psychological therapies and so on, whilst recognising the wellbeing impact of holistic approaches to physical disease interventions. Of course, giving mixed messages is difficult in a written document but much easier in person. We need alignment and coordination of partnerships to ensure a strategic and coordinated approach, and to use the JSNA process to include community assets as well as needs in order to focus on mental wellbeing. By ensuring a single-minded attitude to wellbeing it will be possible to build wellbeing into all existing health and social care agendas.

Mental wellbeing is not expensive but it seems as though there is little appetite for it right now as it may seem costly at a time of austerity. But by tackling more than one item in the list on pages 68–75 we have the chance to offer a value for money argument: more undertaken simultaneously will offer a higher return as a result of the synergy and self-reinforcing savings that accrue. Using the health and wellbeing agenda we can establish a way of removing stigma, and develop a mentally healthy population, including people labelled as mentally ill. QIPP provides an opportunity to set in place a programme that ensures all three of the features we discussed earlier: we can achieve positive mental health for all; we can assist in the prevention of mental illness; and we can offer heightened wellbeing to those living in recovery or with the effects of mental distress.

12.3 Conclusion

The evidence that we have reviewed and the argument that we have developed makes it clear that material circumstances, environmental factors, social context, psychosocial factors, biological factors and behaviours are all important in shaping health and wellbeing, as noted by key reports in this area. This is an ambitious agenda for HWBs, local commissioners, services and communities. In this book we have endeavoured to illustrate the practical steps that can be taken to address this. We don't underestimate the challenge but believe that there is more than ever a good basis on which to act and that positive impacts will be achieved in our lifetimes and for future generations.

Note

1 Public Health Outcomes Framework baseline data included in autumn 2012 publication (DH, 2012a).

Appendix

Bibliography of resources for commissioners

Aked, J., Michaelson, J. and Steuer, N. (2010) *The Role of Local Government in Promoting Wellbeing*. London: Local Government Association Improvement and Development Agency.

Brodie, E., Hughes, T., Jochum, V., Miller, S., Ockenden, N. and Warburton, D. (2011) *Pathways Through Participation: What Creates and Sustains Active Citizenship?* National Council for Voluntary Organisations, Institute for Volunteering Research and Involve. http://pathwaysthroughparticipation.org.uk/resources/finalreport/ (accessed 15 February 2013).

Foresight (2008) *Mental Capital and Wellbeing*. London: Government Office for Science. This presents the findings from a review of the evidence and presents a vision for the opportunities and challenges facing the UK over the next ten years and the implications for everyone's mental wellbeing and mental capital. http://bis.ecgroup.net/Publications/Foresight/MentalCapitalandWellbeing.aspx (accessed 15 February 2013).

Goodspeed, T., Lawlor, E. Neitzert, E. and Nicholls, J. (2009) *A Guide to Social Return on Investment*. Nef. Available at www.neweconomics.org/publications/entry/a-guide-to-social-return-on-investment (accessed 30 June 2013).

Local Government Association has a number of publications that explore local government's new public health role, for example in relation to tackling obesity and alcohol, as well as empowering local communities and engaging people from diverse backgrounds in HealthWatch. www.local.gov.uk/publications (accessed 15 February 2013).

National Institute for Health and Clinical Evidence (NICE) has completed several reviews of interventions to promote population mental wellbeing, or that of sub-populations or specific interventions, which are supported by implementation guidance. www.nice.org.uk/guidance/ (accessed 15 February 2013).

National Mental Wellbeing Impact Assessment (MWIA) Collaborative (2011) *Mental Wellbeing Impact Assessment: A Tooolkit for Well-being, 2011*. Detailed overview of the evidence, population characteristics, determinants and protective factors for mental wellbeing. Describes the process and provides resources for undertaking a MWIA and has a section on measuring wellbeing. www.apho.org.uk/resource/item.aspx?RID=95836 (accessed 15 February 2013).

Nesta (2012) *People Powered Health Co-production Catalogue*. www.nesta.org.uk/library/documents/PPH_v13.pdf (accessed 20 March 2013).

NHS Confederation. Resources for health and wellbeing boards (2012). www.nhsconfed.org/Publications/Pages/lresources-health-wellbeing-boards.aspx (accessed 15 February 2013).

The Poverty Site. This site was monitoring what was happening with regard to poverty and social exclusion in the UK until 2011. Provides poverty related statistics and indicators for different groups. http://poverty.org.uk/ (accessed 15 February 2013).

Social Care online is the UK's largest database of information and research on all aspects of social care and social work. Provides updated daily resources that include legislation, government documents, practice and guidance, systematic reviews, research briefings, reports, journal articles and websites. www.scie-socialcareonline.org.uk/ (accessed 15 February 2013).

The Network of Public Health Observatories produces information, data and intelligence on people's health and health care. The website brings together the national work and products developed by the network of nine PHOs in England (formerly the Association of Public Health Observatories – APHO). Each PHO has a policy lead area and the North East Public Health Observatory (NEPHO) provides access to resources for mental health, but other sites also provide relevant resources. www.apho.org.uk/resource/view.aspx?RID=39436 (accessed 15 February 2013).

References

AACE Diabetes Care Plan Guidelines (2011) *Endocr. Pract.* 17: Suppl. 2.

Abbott, S. and Hobby, L. (2003) 'Who uses welfare benefits advice services in primary care?', *Health and Social Care in the Community*, 11(2): 168–174.

Age Concern and MHF (Mental Health Foundation) (2006) *Promoting Mental Health and Wellbeing in Later Life*.

Aked, J., Michaelson, J., Steuer, N. (2010) *The Role of Local Government in Promoting Wellbeing*. London: Local Government Improvement and Development, nef, and National Mental Health Development Unit.

Ammerman, R. T., Putnam, F. W., Bosse, N. R., Teeters, A. R. and Van Ginkel, J. B. (2010) 'Maternal depression in home visitation: a systematic review', *Aggression and Violent Behaviour*, 15: 191–200.

Andersohn, F., Schade, R., Suissa, S. and Garbe, E. (2009) 'Long-term use of antidepressants for depressive disorders and the risk of diabetes mellitus', *American Journal of Psychiatry*, 166: · 591–598.

Anderson, P., Chisholm, D. and Fuhr, D. C. (2009) 'Effectiveness and cost-effectiveness of policies and programmes to reduce the harm caused by alcohol', *Lancet*, 373: 2234–2246.

Anderson, P., Laurant, M., Kaner, E., Grol, R. and Wensing, M. (2004) 'Engaging general practitioners in the management of alcohol problems: results of a meta-analysis', *Journal of Studies on Alcohol and Drugs*, 65: 191–199.

Anokye, N. K., Trueman, P., Green, C., Pavey, T. G., Hillsdown, M. and Taylor, R. S. (2011) 'The cost-effectiveness of exercise referral schemes', *BMC Public Health*. www.biomedcentral.com/1471-2458/11/9.

Aos, S., Lieb, R., Mayfield, J., Miller, M. and Pennucci, A. (2004) *Benefits and Costs of Prevention and Early Intervention Programs for Youth*. Washington, DC: Washington State Institute for Public Policy.

Appleby, L., Warner, R., Whitton, A. and Faragher, B. (1997) 'A controlled study of fluoxetine and cognitive-behavioural counselling in the treatment of postnatal depression', *British Medical Journal*, 314(932): 936.

Arbelaez, J. J., Ariyo, A. A., Crum, R. M., Fried, L. P. and Ford, D. E. (2007) 'Depressive symptoms, inflammation, and ischemic stroke in older adults: a prospective analysis in the cardiovascular health study', *Journal of the American Geriatrics Society*, 55: 1825–1830.

Armstrong, K. L. and Morris, J. (2000) 'Promoting secure attachment, maternal mood and child health in a vulnerable population: a randomized controlled trial', *Journal of Paediatrics and Child Health*, 36(6): 555–562.

Arnstein, S. R. A. (1969) 'Ladder of citizen participation', *Journal of the American Institute of Planners*, 35(4): 216–224.

Askey-Jones, S. (2009) *Enhancing the mental well-being of people with multiple sclerosis*. London: Nursing Times.

Askey-Jones, S., Silber, E., Shaw, P., Gray, R. and David, A.S. (2012) 'A nurse-led mental health service for people with multiple sclerosis', *Journal of Psychosomatic Research* 72: 463–465.

Barlow, J. et al. (2003) 'Parent training programs for improving maternal psychosocial health', *Cochrane Database of Systematic Reviews*, Issue 4.

Barlow, J. and Coren, E. (2004) 'Parent-training programmes for improving maternal psychosocial health', *Cochrane Database of Systematic Reviews*, 1.

Barlow, J., Kirkpatrick, S., Wood, D., Ball, M. and Stewart-Brown, S. (2007a) *Family and Parenting Support in Sure Start Local Programmes. National Evaluation of Sure Start*. London: Birkbeck College, London University.

Barlow, J. et al. (2007b) 'The Oxfordshire Home Visitation Study', in J. Beecham and I. Sinclair (2007) *Costs and Outcomes in Children's Social Care*, London: Jessica Kingsley.

Barker, I., and Peck, E. (eds) (1987) *Power In Strange Places: User Empowerment in Mental Health Services*. London: Good Practices in Mental Health.

Barrett, H. (2010), *The Delivery of Parent Skills Training Programmes: Meta-analytic Studies and Systematic Reviews of What Works Best*. London: Family and Parenting Institute.

Barry, M., Domitrovich, C. and Lara, M. A. (2005) 'The implementation of mental health promotion programmes', *Promotion and Education* (Suppl.), 2: 30–36.

Barry, M. and Friedli, L. (2008) *The Influence of Social, Demographic and Physical Factors on Positive Mental Health in Children, Adults and Older People*. London: State-of-Science Review: SR-B3.

Barry, M. and Jenkins, R. (2006) *Implementing Mental Health Promotion: A Practical Guide to Planning, Implementing and Evaluating Mental Health Promotion Programmes*. Edinburgh: Churchill Livingstone.

Barry, M. and Jenkins, R. (2007) *Implementing Mental Health Promotion*. Philadelphia: Elsevier.

Barth, J., Schumacher, M. and Herrmann-Lingen, C. (2004) 'Depression as a risk factor for mortality in patients with coronary heart disease: a meta-analysis', *Psychosomatic Medicine*, 66(6): 802–813.

Bayatpour, M., Wells, R. and Holford, S. (1992) 'Physical and sexual abuse as predictors of substance use and suicide among pregnant teenagers', *Journal of Adolescent Health*, 13(2): 128–132.

Belippa, J. (1991) *Illness or Distress? Alternative Models of Mental Health*. London: Confederation of Indian Organisations.

Bell, J. T. and Spector, T. D. (2011) 'A twin approach to unravelling epigenetics', *Trends in Genetics*, 27(3): 116–125.

Bellis, M., Lowey, H., Hughes, K., Deacon, L. and Perkins, C. (2012) 'Variations in risk and protective factors for life satisfaction and mental wellbeing with deprivation: a cross-sectional study', *BMC Public Health*, 12(1): 492–508.

Belsky, J., Melhuish, E., Barnes, J. et al. (2006) 'Effect of Sure Start local programmes on children and families: early findings from a quasi-experimental, cross-sectional study', *British Medical Journal*, 332: 1476–1478.

Ben-Shlomo, Y. and Kuh, D. (2002) 'A life course approach to chronic disease epidemiology: conceptual models, empirical challenges and interdisciplinary perspectives', *International Journal of Epidemiology*, 31(285): 293.

Bennett, A., Appleton, X. and Jackson, C. (2011) *Practical Mental Health Commissioning: A Framework for Local Authority and NHS Commissioners of Mental Health and Wellbeing Services*. London: Royal College of Psychiatrists.

Bentley, C. (2007) *Addressing Health Inequalities – From Mystery and Imagination to Practical Action*. Powerpoint presentation. Health Inequalities National Support Team.

Binder, M. and Coad, A. (2010) 'An examination of the dynamics of well-being and life events using vector autoregressions', *Journal of Economic Behavior and Organization*, 76: 352–371.

Black, C. (2008) *Working for a Healthier Tomorrow*. London: Department of Health.

Blake, G., Diamond, J., Foot, J., Gidley, B., Mayo, M., Shukra, K. and Yarnit, M. (2008) *Community Engagement and Community Cohesion*. York: Joseph Rowntree.

Blas, E. and Kurup, S. (2010) *Equity, Social Determinants and Public Health Programmes*. Geneva: World Health Organization.

Blumethal, J. A. (2007) 'Psychosocial training and cardiac rehabilitation', *Journal of Cardiopulmonary Rehabilitation*, 27(2): 104–106.

Boden, J. M., Horwood, L. J. and Fergusson, D. M. (2007) 'Exposure to childhood sexual and physical abuse and subsequent educational achievement outcomes', *Child Abuse and Neglect*, 31(10): 1101–1114.

Boehm J. K., Kubzansky L. D. (2012) 'The heart's content: the association between positive psychological well-being and cardiovascular health', *Psychol Bull.*, 138(4):655–91.

Boehm, J. K., Peterson, C., Kivimaki, M. and Kubzansky, L. (2011) 'A prospective study of positive psychological well-being and coronary heart disease', *Health Psychology*, 30(3): 259–267.

Bond, L., Carlin, J. B., Rubin, K. and Patton, G. (2001) 'Does bullying cause emotional problems? A prospective study of young teenagers', *British Medical Journal*, 323: 480–484.

Bond, L., Mason, P., Tannahill, C., Egan, M. and Whitely, E. (2012) 'Exploring the relationships between housing, neighbourhoods and mental wellbeing for residents of deprived areas', *BMC Public Health*, 12: 48.

Bond, L., Patton, G., Carlin, J. B., Butler, H., Thomas, L. and Bowes, G. (2004) 'The Gatehouse Project: can a multi-level school intervention affect emotional wellbeing and health risk behaviours', *Journal of Epidemiology and Community Health*, 58: 997–1003.

Bonin, E.-M., Stevens, M., Beecham, J., Byford, S. and Parsonage, M. (2011) 'Costs and longer-term savings of parenting programmes for the prevention of persistent conduct disorder: a modelling study', *BMC Public Health*, 11: 803.

Bornemisza, O., Ransom, M. K., Poletti, T. M. and Sondorp, E. (2010) 'Promoting health equity in conflict-affected fragile states', *Social Science and Medicine*, 70: 80–88.

Bourdel-Marchasson, I., Mouries, A. and Helmer, C. (2010) 'Hyperglycaemia, microangiopathy, diabetes and dementia risk', *Diabetes and Metabolism*, 36 (Suppl. 3): 112–118.

Brayne, C., Gaob, L. and Matthews, F. (2005) 'Challenges in the epidemiological investigation of the relationships between physical activity, obesity, diabetes, dementia and depression', *Neurobiology of Aging*, 26S: S6–S10.

Brodie, E., Hughes, T., Jochum, V., Miller, S., Ockenden, N. and Warburton, D. (2011) *Pathways Through Participation: What Creates and Sustains Active Citizenship?* London: National Council for Voluntary Organisations, Institute for Volunteering Research and Involve. http://pathwaysthroughparticipation.org.uk/resources/finalreport/ (accessed 15 February 2013).

Brookoff, D., O'Brien, K. K., Cook, C. S., Thompson, T. D. and Williams, C. (1997) 'Characteristics of participants in domestic violence assessment at the scene of domestic assault', *JAMA*, 277(17): 1369–1373.

Brown, S. and Taylor, K. (2008) 'Bullying, education and earnings: evidence from the National Child Development Study', *Economics of Education Review*, 27: 387–401.

Burns, R.A. and Machina, M.A. (2010) 'Identifying gender differences in the independent effects of personality and psychological well-being on two broad affect components of subjective well-being', *Personality and Individual Differences*, 48 (1): 22–27.

Burton, A. and Hitch, B. (2012) *Improving Mental Well-Being in Oxfordshire (2009–2012).* Oxford: Oxfordshire PCT.

Burton, E. J., Mitchell, L. and Stride, C. B. (2011) 'Good places for ageing in place: development of objective built environment measures for investigating links with older people's wellbeing', *BMC Public Health*, 11: 839.

Busfield, J. (1996) *Men, Women and Madness.* New York: NYU.

Bywater, T., Hutchings, J., Daley, D. and Whitaker, C. (2009) 'Long-term effectiveness of a parenting intervention for children at risk of developing conduct disorder', *British Journal of Psychiatry*, 195: 318–324.

Caan, W. and Jenkins, R. (2009) 'Integrating the promotion of child mental health into national policies for health sector reform', *Journal of Public Health*, 7(1): 9–14.

Cabinet Office (2006) *Reaching Out: An Action Plan on Social Exclusion.* http://webarchive.nationalarchives.gov.uk/20070705125957/cabinetoffice.gov.uk/social_exclusion_task_force/publications/reaching_out/ (accessed 25 March 2013).

Campion, J. (2009) 'Economics of interventions: a draft of the evidence', personal communication.

Campayo, A.D., de Jonge, P., Roy, J.F., Saz, P., de la Cámara, C., Quintanilla, M.A., Marcos, G., Ãirbara, J. S. and Lobo, A. (2010) 'Depressive Disorder and Incident Diabetes Mellitus: The Effect of Characteristics of Depression', *Am J Psychiatry*, 167:580–588.

Campayo, A., Gomez-Biel, C.H. and Lobo, A. (2011) 'Diabetes and Depression', *Curr. Psychiatry Rep*, 13:26–30.

Campion, J. and Nurse, J. (2007) 'A dynamic model for wellbeing', *Australasian Psychiatry*, 15(S1): 24–28.

Canning, D. and Bowser, D. (2010) 'Investing in health to improve the wellbeing of the disadvantaged: reversing the argument of *Fair Society, Healthy Lives (The Marmot Review)*', *Social Science and Medicine*, 71: 1223–1226.

Carroll, C., Patterson, M., Wood, S., Booth, A., Rick, J. and Balain, J. (2007) 'A conceptual framework for implementation fidelity', *Implementation Science*, 2: 40.

Carter, S. M., Rychetnik, R., Lloyd, B., Kerridge, I. H., Baur, L., Bauman, A., Hooker, C. and Zask, A. (2011) 'Evidence, ethics, and values: a framework for health promotion', *American Journal of Public Health*, 101(3): 465–472.

Carver, C. S., Scheier, M. F. and Segerstrom, S. C. (2010) 'Optimism', *Clinical Psychology Review*, 30(7): 879–889.

Casiday, R., Kinsman, E., Fisher, C. and Bambra, C. (2008) *Volunteering and Health: What Impact Does It Really Have?* London: Volunteering England.

Certain, H. E., Mueller, M., Jagodzinski, T. and Fleming, M. (2008) 'Domestic abuse during the previous year in a sample of postpartum women', *Journal of Obstetric, Gynecologic, and Neonatal Nursing*, 37(1): 35–41.

Chan, N., Ho, D., Ho, W.-L. et al. (2007) *The Needs of Chinese Older People with Dementia and their Carers*. Manchester: Wai Yin Chinese Women Society.

Chana, W., McCraeb, R. R., Rogers, D. L., Weimer, A. A., Greenberg, D. M. and Terracciano, A. (2011) 'Rater wealth predicts perceptions of outgroup competence', *Journal of Research in Personality*, 45(6): 597–603.

Chen, H.-T. (1990) *Theory-Driven Evaluations*. London: Sage Publications.

Cheng, S.-T. and Chan, A. C. (2005) 'Measuring psychological well-being in the Chinese', *Personality and Individual Differences*, 38(6): 1307–1316.

Chick, J., Lloyd, G. and Crombie, E. (1985) 'Counselling problem drinkers in medical wards: a controlled study', *BMJ*, 290, 965–967.

Chisholm, D., Rehm, J., van Ommeren, M. and Monteiro, M. (2004) 'Reducing the global burden of hazardous alcohol use: a comparative and cost effectiveness analysis', *Journal of Studies on Alcohol*, 65(6): 782–793

Clark, F., Jackson, J., Carlson, M., Chou, C.-P., Cherry, B. J., Fordan-Marsh, M., Knight, B. G., Mandel, D., Blanchard, J., Granger, D. A., Wilcox, R. R., Lai, M. Y., White, B., Hay, J., Lam, C., Martella, A. and Azen, S. P. (2012) 'Effectiveness of a lifestyle intervention in promoting the well-being of independently living older people: results of the Well Elderly 2 Randomised Controlled Trial', *Journal of Epidemiology and Community Health*, 66(9): 782–790.

Cobden, D. S., Niessen, L. W., Barr, C. E., Rutten, F. F. H. and Redekop, K. (2010) 'Relationships among self-management, patient perceptions of care, and health economic outcomes for decision-making and clinical practice in Type 2 diabetes', *International Society for Pharmacoeconomics and Outcomes Research (ISPOR)*, 13(1): 138–147.

Cohen, J. A., Mannarino, A. P. and Iyengar, S. (2011) 'Community treatment of posttraumatic stress disorder for children exposed to intimate partner violence: a randomized controlled trial', *Archives of Pediatrics & Adolescent Medicine*, 165(1): 16–21.

Cooper, P. J., Murray, L., Wilson, A. and Romaniuk, H. (2003) 'Controlled trial of the short- and long-term effect of psychological treatment of post-partum depression. I. Impact on maternal mood', *British Journal of Psychiatry*, 182: 412–419.

Cornah, D. (2004) 'Promoting engagement: identifying why effective early interventions for children with/or at risk of developing mental health problems sometimes fail to reach them most', *Journal of the American Medical Association*, 278(8): 637–643.

Cornah, D., Sonuga-Barke, E., Stevenson, J. and Thompson, M. (2003) 'The impact of maternal mental health and child's behavioural difficulties on attributions about child behaviour', *British Journal of Clinical Psychology*, 42(1): 69–79.

Costa, P.T., Jr. and McCrae, R.R. (1992). Revised NEO Personality Inventory (NEO-PI-R) and NEO Five-Factor Inventory (NEO-FFI) manual. Odessa, FL: Psychological Assessment Resources.

Costa, P.T. and Robert R. McCrae, R.R. (1990). 'Personality Disorders and The Five-Factor Model of Personality', *Journal of Personality Disorders*, 4 (4): 362–371.

Coulter, A. (2009) *Engaging Communities for Health Improvement: A Scoping Study for the Health Foundation*. London: Health Foundation.

Cross, T. P., Mathews, B., Tonmyr, L., Scott, D. and Ouimet, C. (2012) 'Child welfare policy and practice on children's exposure to domestic violence', *Child Abuse and Neglect*, 36(3), 210–216.

Cross, W. and West, J. (2011) 'Examining implementer fidelity: conceptualising and measuring adherence and competence', *Journal of Children's Services*, 6(1): 18–33.

Cuijpers, P., Riper, H. and Lemmers, L. (2004) 'The effects on mortality of brief interventions for problem drinking: a meta-analysis', *Addiction*, 99:839–45.

Cukierman, T., Gerstien, H. C. and Williamson, J. D. (2005) 'Cognitive decline and dementia in diabetes: systematic overview of prospective observational studies', *Diabetologia*, 48: 2460–2469.

Damschroder, L.J., Aron, D.C., Keith, R.E., Kirsh, S.R., Alexander, J.A., Lowery, J.C. (2009) 'Fostering implementation of health services research findings into practice: a consolidated framework for advancing implementation science', *Implementation Science*. 4:50.

Danna, K. and Griffin, R. W. (1999) 'Health and well-being in the workplace: a review and synthesis of the literature', *Journal of Management*, 25(3): 357–384.

Davidson, K. W. (2011) 'Depression and comorbid coronary heart disease', *Medscape Education Psychiatry and Mental Health*, www.medscape.org/viewarticle/749924 (accessed 25 March 2013).

Davies, J. K. and Sherriff, N. (2011) 'The gradient in health inequalities among families and children: a review of evaluation frameworks', *Health Policy*, 101: 1–10.

Davies, J. K. and Sherriff, N. (2012) *The Gradient Evaluation Framework*. Brighton, UK: University of Brighton.

Deeg, D. J. and Thomese, G. (2005) 'Discrepancies between personal income and neighbourhood status: effects on physical and mental health', *European Journal on Ageing*, 2(2): 98–108.

de Groot, M., Dyle, T., Kushnick, M., Shubrook, J., Merrill, J., Rabideau, E. and Schwartz, F. (2012) 'Can lifestyle interventions do more than reduce diabetes risk? Treating depression in adults with type 2 diabetes with exercise and cognitive behavioral therapy', *Current Diabetes Reports*, 12: 157–166.

de Hert, M., Dekker, J. M., Kahl, K. G., Holt, R. I. and Moller, H. J. (2009) 'Cardiovascular disease and diabetes in people with severe mental illness position statement from the European Psychiatric Association (EPA), supported by the European Association for the Study of Diabetes (EASD) and the European Society of Cardiology (ESC)', *European Psychiatry*, 24(6): 412–424.

DH (Department of Health) (2004) *Alcohol Needs Assessment Research Project (ANARP): The 2004 National Alcohol Needs Assessment for England*. London: HM Government.

DH (Department of Health) (2009a) *New Horizons: A shared vision for mental health*. London: HM Government.

DH (Department of Health) (2009b) *NHS Health and Wellbeing: Final Report*. London: HM Government.

DH (Department of Health) (2009c) *Health and Wellbeing at Work in the United Kingdom*. London: HM Government.

DH (Department of Health) (2010) *Responding to Violence Against Women and Children – the Role of the NHS: The Report of the Taskforce on the Health Aspects of Violence Against Women and Children*. London: Department of Health.

DH (Department of Health) (2011a) *NHS Outcomes Framework 2012–13*. London: Department of Health.

DH (Department of Health) (2011b) Public Health in Local Government. London: Department of Health.

DH (Department of Health) (2012a) *Improving Outcomes and Supporting Transparency. Part 1: A Public Health Outcomes Framework for England, 2013–2016.* London: Department of Health.

DH (Department of Health) (2012b) *Local Healthwatch: A Strong Voice for Local People – the Policy Explained.* London: Department of Health.

DH (Department of Health) (2013a) *Commissioning Framework for Health and Wellbeing.* London: Department of Health.

DH (Department of Health) (2013b) *Healthy Lives, Healthy People: Consultation on the Funding and Commissioning Routes for Public Health Launch Date.* London: Department of Health.

Diabetes UK (2010) *Emotional and Psychological Support and Care in Diabetes.* London: Diabetes UK.

Dickens, A. P., Richards, S. H., Hawton, A., Taylor, R. S., Greaves, C. J., Green, C., Edwards, R. and Campbell, J. L. (2011) 'An evaluation of the effectiveness of a community mentoring service for socially isolated older people: a controlled trial', *BMC Public Health*, 11(1): 218–231.

Diener, E. (1984) 'Subjective well-being', *Psychological Bulletin*, 95(3): 542–575.

Diener, E. (2000) 'Subjective well-being: The science of happiness, and a proposal for national index', *American Psychologist*, 55: 34–43.

Diener, E. and Chan, M. Y. (1984) 'Happy people live longer: subjective well-being contributes to health and longevity', *Applied Psychology: Health and Well-Being*, 3: 1–43.

Diener, E., Suh, E. M., Lucas, R. E. and Smith, H. L. (1999) 'Subjective well-being: three decades of progress', *Psychological Bulletin*, 125(2): 276–302.

Drummond, C., Phillips, T., Coulton, S., Barnaby, B., Keating, S., Sabri, R. and Moloney, J. (2003) *Saturday Night and Sunday Morning: The 2003 Twenty-four Hour National Prevalence Survey of Alcohol-related Attendances at Accident and Emergency Departments in England.* Department of Health, unpublished research report to the Strategy Unit.

Eaton, W.W., Armenian, H., Gallo, J., Pratt, L., and Ford, D. E. (1996) 'Depression and risk for onset of type II diabetes: a prospective population-based study', *Diabetes Care*, 19(10): 1097–1102.

Edge D. (2007) 'Ethnicity, psychosocial risk, and perinatal depression–a comparative study among inner-city women in the United Kingdom', *J Psychosom Res.*, 63(3):291–5.

Edwards, R. T., Ceilleachair, A., Bywater, T., Hughes, A. and Hutchings, J. (2007) 'Parenting programme for parents of children at risk of developing conduct disorder: cost effectiveness analysis', *British Medical Journal*, 334: 682.

Egan, M., Tannahill, C., Petticrew, M. and Thomas, S. (2008) 'Psychosocial risk factors in home and community settings and their associations with population health and health inequalities: a systematic meta-review', *BMC Public Health*, 8: 239.

Egede, L. E., Nietert, P. J. and Zheng, D. (2005) 'Depression and all-cause and coronary heart disease mortality among adults with and without diabetes', *Diabetes Care*, 28: 1339–1345.

Elasy, T. (2010) 'Type 2 diabetes prevention: an opportunity for a new discipline', *Clinical Diabetes*, 28(2): 49–50.

Erskine, S., Maheswaran, R., Pearson, T. and Gleeson, D. (2010) 'Socioeconomic deprivation, urban-rural location and alcohol-related mortality in England and Wales', *BMC Public Health*, 10:99.

Esping-Andersen, G. (2007) 'More inequality and fewer opportunities? Structural determinants and human agency in the dynamics of income distribution', in D. Held and A. Kaya (eds), *Global Inequality*. Cambridge: Polity Press, pp. 216–251.

Etnier, J. L., Salazar, W., Landers, D. M., Petruzzello, S. J., Han, M. and Nowell, P. (1997) 'The influence of physical fitness and exercise upon cognitive functioning: a meta-analysis', *Journal of Sport and Exercise Psychology (JSEP)*, 19(3): 249–277.

Evans, G. W. (2004) 'The environment of childhood poverty', *American Psychologist*, 59(2): 77–92.

Evans, G. W. and Kim, P. (2007) 'Childhood poverty and health: cumulative risk exposure and stress dysregulation', *Psychological Science*, 18(11): 953–957.

Evers, K.E., Prochaska, J.O., Van Marter, D.F., Johnson, J.L. and Prochaska, J.M. (2007). 'Transtheoretical-based bullying prevention effectiveness trials in middle schools and high schools, *Educational Research*, 49, 397–414.

Fals-Stewart, W. (2003) 'The occurrence of partner physical aggression on days of alcohol consumption: a longitudinal diary study', *Journal of Consulting and Clinical Psychology*, 71: 41–52.

Fennell, M. J. V. (2009) *Overcoming Low Self-Esteem*. London: Constable and Robinson.

Ferdinand, K. C., Orenstein, D., Hong, Y., Journigan, J. G., Trogdon, J., Bowman, J., Zohrabian, A., Kilgore, M., White, A., Mokdad, A., Pechacek, T. F., Goetzel, R. Z., Labarthe, D. R., Puckrein, G. A., Finkelstein, E., Wang, G., French, M. E. and Vaccarino, V. (2011) 'Health economics of cardiovascular disease: defining the research', *CVD Prevention and Control*, 6: 91–100.

Fergusson, D. M., Boden, J. M. and Horwood, L. J. (2008) 'Exposure to childhood sexual and physical abuse and adjustment in early adulthood', *Child Abuse and Neglect*, 32: 607–619.

Field, T. (2011) 'Prenatal depression effects on early development: a review', *Infant Behavior and Development*, 34: 1–14.

Fischer, R. and Boer, D. (2011) 'What is more important for national well-being: money or autonomy? A meta-analysis of well-being, burnout, and anxiety across 63 societies', *Journal of Personality and Social Psychology*, 10(1): 164–184.

Fixsen, D.L. and Blase, K.A. (2009) Implementation: the missing link between research and practice', NIRN Implementation Brief 1.Available at: http://caps.ucsf.edu (accessed 21 June 2013).

Fixsen, D. L., Naoom, S. F., Blase, K. A., Friedman, R. M. and Wallace, F. (2005) *Implementation Research: A Synthesis of the Literature*. Miami, FL: National Implementation Research Network at the Louis de la Parte Florida Mental Health Institute, University of South Florida.

Fleming, M. F., Manwell, L. B., Barry, K. L., Adams, W. And Stauffacher, E. A. (1999) 'Brief physician advice for alcohol problems in older adults: a randomized community-based trial, *Journal of Family Practice*, 48: 378–484.

Forrester, D. and Harwin, J. (2010) *Parents Who Misuse Drugs and Alcohol: Effective Interventions in Social Work and Child Protection*. Chichester: Wiley.

Foresight (2008) *Mental Capital and Wellbeing*. London: Government Office for Science.

Fowler, P.J., Tompsett, C.J., Braciszewski, J.M., Jacques-Tiura, A.J. Baltes, B.B. (2009) 'Community violence: a meta-analysis on the effect of exposure and mental health outcomes of children and adolescents', *Development and Psychopathology*, 21: 227–25.

Fraser, N., and Honneth, A. (1997) 'Redistribution or Recognition? A Political-philosophical Exchange. London: Verso.

Frasure-Smith, N. and Lesperance, F. (2005) 'Depression and coronary heart disease: complex synergism of mind, body, and environment', *Current Directions in Psychological Science*, 14(1): 39–43.

Friedli, L. (2003). *Making it Effective: A Guide to Evidence Based Mental Health Promotion*. London: Centre for Mental Health.

Friedli, L. (2009) *Mental Health, Resilience and Inequalities*. Copenhagen: WHO Europe.

Friedli, L., Jackson, C., Abernethy, H. and Stansfield, J. (2008) *Social Prescribing for Mental Health – A Guide to Commissioning and Delivery*. London and Manchester: CSIP/NWDC.

Friedli, L. and Parsonage, M. (2007) *Mental Health Promotion: Building an Economic Case*. Belfast: Northern Ireland Association for Mental Health.

Friel, S. and Marmot, M.G. (2011) 'Action on the Social Determinants of Health and Health Inequities Goes Global', *Annual Review of Public Health*, 32: 225–36.

Fulford, K. W. M. (2004) 'Facts/values: ten principles of values-based medicine', in J. Radden (ed.) *The Philosophy of Psychiatry: A Companion*. New York: Oxford University Press, pp. 205–234.

Fulford, K. W. M., Peile, E. and Carroll, H. (2012) *Essential Values-Based Practice: Clinical Stories linking Science with People*. Cambridge: Cambridge University Press.

Gale, C. R., Dennison, E. M., Cooper, C. and Sayer, A. A. (2011) 'Neighbourhood environment and positive mental health in older people: the Hertfordshire Cohort Study', *Health and Place*, 17: 867–874 .

Gallagher, M. W., Lopez, S. J. and Preacher, K. J. (2009) 'The hierarchical structure of well-being', *Journal of Personality*, 77: 1025–10.

Garcia, D. (2011) 'Two models of personality and well-being among adolescents', *Personality and Individual Differences*, 50(8): 1208–1212.

Gardner, F., Burton, J. and Klimes, I. (2006) 'Randomised controlled trial of a parenting intervention in the voluntary sector: outcomes and mechanism for change', *Journal of Child Psychology and Psychiatry*, 47: 1123–1132.

Gillies, C. L., Abrams, K. R., Lambert, P. C., Cooper, N. J., Sutton, A. J., Hsu, R.T. and Khunti, K. (2007) 'Pharmacological and lifestyle interventions to prevent or delay type 2 diabetes in people with impaired glucose tolerance: systematic review and meta-analysis', *BMJ*, doi:10.1136/bmj.39063.689375.55. 2007.

Giltay, E. J., Geleijnse, J. M., Zitman, F. G., Buijsse, B. and Kromhout, D. (2007) 'Lifestyle and dietary correlates of dispositional optimism in men: the Zutphen Elderly Study', *Journal of Psychosomatic Research*, 63: 483–490.

Giltay E. J., Kamphuis M. H., Kalmijn S., Zitman F. G., Kromhout D. (2006) 'Dispositional optimism and the risk of cardiovascular death: the Zutphen Elderly Study', *Arch Intern Med.*, 166(4):431–6.

Giltay, E. J., Zitman, F. G., Kromhout, D. (2006) 'Dispositional optimism and the risk of depressive symptoms during 15 years of follow-up: the Zutphen Elderly Study', *J Affect Disord.*, 91(1):45–52.

Glover, G., Lee, R. and Copeland, A. (2010) *The Development of a Prototype Index of Ecological Factors Affecting Wellbeing in the Population*. Stockton, Teeside: North East Public Health Observatory.

Glover, V. and O'Connor, T. G. (2002) 'Effects of antenatal stress and anxiety: implications for development and psychiatry', *British Journal of Psychiatry*, 180: 389–391.

Gonzalez, J.S., Safren, S.A., Cagliero, E., Wexler, D.J., Delahanty, L., Wittenberg, E., Blais, M. A., Meigs, J. B. and Grant, R. W. (2007) 'Depression, self-care, and medication adherence in type 2 diabetes: relationships across the full range of symptom severity', *Diabetes Care*, 30(9): 2222–2227.

Goodman, A., Joyce, R. and Smith, J. P. (2011) 'The long shadow cast by childhood physical and mental problems on adult life', *Proceedings of the National Academy of Sciences of the United States of America*, 108(15): 6032–6037.

Goodspeed, T., Lawlor, E., Neitzert, E. and Nicholls, J. (2009) *A Guide to Social Return on Investment*. Nef. Online resource. Available at: http://www.neweconomics.org/publications/entry/a-guide-to-social-return-on-investment (accessed 30 June 2013).

Greasley, P. and Small, N. (2005) 'Providing welfare advice in general practice: referrals, issues and outcomes', *Health and Social Care in the Community*, 13(3): 249–258.

Greene, R., Pugh, R., Roberts, D. (2008) 'Black and minority ethnic parents with mental health problems and their children'. Research briefing 29, London: Social Care Institute for Excellence (SCIE).

Gribble, K. D. (2006) 'Mental health, attachment and breastfeeding: implications for adopted children and their mothers', *International Breastfeeding Journal*, 1: 5.

Grime, P. R. (2004) 'Computerised cognitive behavioural therapy at work: a randomized controlled trial in employees with recent stress related absenteeism', *Occupational Medicine*, 54(5): 353–359.

Grynszpan, D. et al. (2010) *International Dimensions of Climate Change*. London: Government Office for Science: Foresight Report.

Halfon, N. and Hochstein, M. (2002) 'Life course health development: an integrated framework for developing health, policy, and research', *Milbank Quarterly*, 80(3): 422–479.

Halfon, N., Russ, S. and Ragaldo, M. (2005) *The Life Course Health Development Model: A Guide to Children's Health Care Policy and Practice*. Zero to Three.

Hamer, M. and Chida, Y. (2008) 'Walking and primary prevention: a meta-analysis of prospective cohort studies', *British Journal of Sports Medicine*, 42: 238–243.

Hart, S., Fonareva, I., Merluzzi, N. and Mohr, D. C. (2005) 'Treatment for depression and its relationship to improvement in quality of life and psychological well-being in multiple sclerosis patients', *Quality of Life Research*, 14: 695–703.

Harvey, S. B., Hotopf, M., Overland, S. and Mykletun, A. (2010) 'Physical activity and common mental disorders', *British Journal of Psychiatry*, 197: 357–364.

Hawe, P., Shiell, A., Riley, T. and Gold, L. (2004) 'Methods for exploring implementation variation and local context within a randomised community intervention trial', *Journal of Epidemiology and Community Health*, 58: 788–793.

Hawkins, N. M., Jhund, P. S., McMurray, J. J. V. and Capewell, S. (2012) 'Socioeconomic deprivation is a powerful independent predictor of HF development and adverse outcomes', *European Journal of Heart Failure*, 14: 138–146.

Hay, D. F., Pawlby, S., Angold, A., Harold, G. T. and Sharp, D. (2003) 'Pathways to violence in the children of mothers who were depressed postpartum', *Developmental Psychology*, 39: 1083–1094.

Heginbotham, C. (2012) *Values-Based Commissioning of Health and Social Care*. Cambridge: Cambridge University Press.

Heikkilä, K., Sacker, A., Kelly, Y., Renfrew, M. J. and Quigley, M. A. (2011) 'Breast feeding and child behaviour in the Millennium Cohort Study', *Archives of Disease in Childhood*, 96(7): 635–642.

Herron, S. and Mortimer, R. (1999) 'Mental health: a contested concept', *Journal of Public Mental Health*, 1(1): 4–8.

Herron, S. and Trent, D. (2000) 'Mental health: a secondary concept to mental illness', *Journal of Public Mental Health*, 2(2): 29–38.

Hex, N., Bartlett, C., Wright, D., Taylor, M. and Varley, D. (2012) 'Estimating the current and future costs of Type 1 and Type 2 diabetes in the UK, including direct health costs and indirect societal and productivity costs', *Diabetic Medicine*, 29 (7): 855–862.

Hilton, M. (2005) *Assessing the Financial Return on Investment of Good Management Strategies and the WORC Project*. Queensland, Australia: WORC.

HM Government (2005) *Health, Work and Well-being – Caring for our Future*, www.dwp.gov.uk/docs/health-and-wellbeing.pdf (accessed 20 March 2013).

HM Government (2012) *Health and Social Care Act 2012*. London: HM Government.

HM Government/Department of Health (2011) *No Health Without Mental Health: A Cross-Government Mental Health Outcomes Strategy for People of All Ages*. London: Department of Health.

Hopper, K. (2007) 'Rethinking social recovery in schizophrenia: what a capabilities approach might offer', *Social Science and Medicine*, 65(5): 868–879.

Howarth, J. (2012) 'Developing Cumbria Partnership Foundation Trust as a Public Health Organisation'. Carlisle: Cumbria Partnership NHS Foundation Trust.

Hummel, S., Blank, L., Goyder, L., Guillame, L., Wilkinson, A. and Chilcott, J. (2009) *Draft Systematic Review of the Effectiveness of Universal Interventions which Aim to Promote Emotional and Social Wellbeing in Secondary Schools*. Sheffield: SCHARR, University of Sheffield.

Hunter, C. (2011) *Responding to Children and Young People's Disclosures of Abuse*. Australian Institute of Family Studies. NCPC practice brief: National Child Protection Clearing House, Melbourne, Australia.

Innes, A., Macpherson, S., McCabe, L. (2006) *Promoting Person-Centred Care at the Front Line*. York: Joseph Rowntree Foundation.

Ismail K., Lawrence-Smith G., Cheah Y., Winkley K., Yadav R., Thomas S., Bartlett J. (2009) 'Motivational enhancement therapy with and without CBT to treat type 1 diabetes: the long-term outcomes of a randomized controlled trial', *Diabetologia*. 52:s14–s14.

Itzin, C. (2006) *Tackling the Health and Mental Health Effects of Domestic and Sexual Violence and Abuse*. London: Department of Health. Accessed at www.dh.gov.uk/en/Publicationsandstatistic

Itzin, C., Bailey, S., Bentovim, A. (2008) 'The effects of domestic violence and sexual abuse on mental health', *The Psychiatrist*, 32: 448–450.

Jonas, W. (2005) *Mosby's Dictionary of Complementary and Alternative Medicine*. Philadelphia: Elsevier.

Jones, L., James, M., Jefferson, T., Lushey, C., Morleo, M., Stokes, E., Sumnall, H., Witty, K. and Bellis, M. (2007) *Alcohol and Schools: A Review of the Effectiveness and Cost-effectiveness of*

Interventions Delivered in Primary and Secondary Schools to Prevent and/or Reduce Alcohol Use by Young People Under 18 Years Old. Final Report. Centre for Public Health, Liverpool John Moores University. PHIAC 14.3a. www.nice.org.uk/nicemedia/pdf/AlcoholSchoolsConsReview. pdf (accessed 2 March 2008).

Joseph, S. and Wood, A. (2010) 'Assessment of positive functioning in clinical psychology: theoretical and practical issues', *Clinical Psychology Review*, 30(7): 830–838.

Joseph Rowntree Foundation (2005) *The Older People's Inquiry: 'That Little Bit of Help'*. York: Joseph Rowntree Foundation. Online resource. Available at: www.jrf.org.uk/sites/files/jrf/ briefing03.pdf (accessed 1 July 2013).

Kaner, E. F., Beyer, F., Dickinson, H. O., Pienaar, E., Campbell, F., Schlesinger, C., Heather, N., Saunders, J. and Burnand, B. (2007) 'Effectiveness of brief alcohol interventions in primary care populations', *Cochrane Database of Systematic Reviews*, 18(2).

Karam, J. G. and McFarlane, S. I. (2011) 'Update on the prevention of Type 2 diabetes', *Current Diabetes Reports*, 11: 56–63.

Karoly, L., Kilburn, M. R. and Cannon, J. (2005) *Early Childhood Interventions: Proven Results, Future Promise*. Santa Monica, CA: Rand Corporation.

Kashdan, T. B., Biswas-Diener, R. and King, L. A. (2008) 'Reconsidering happiness: The costs of distinguishing between hedonics and eudaimonia', *Journal of Positive Psychology*, 3(4): 219–233.

Kashdan, T. B. and Rottenberg, J. (2010) 'Psychological flexibility as a fundamental aspect of health', *Clinical Psychology Review*, 30(7): 865–887.

Kasper, D. L., Braunwald, E. and Fauci, A. (2005) *Harrison's Principles of Internal Medicine* (16th edn). New York: McGraw-Hill.

Katon, W., Unutzer, J., Fan, M.-Y., Williams, J. W., Scoenbaum, M., Lin, E. H. B. and Hunkeler, E. M. (2006) 'Cost-effectiveness and net benefit of enhanced treatment of depression for older adults with diabetes and depression', *Diabetes Care*, 29: 265–270.

Kendrick, D., Elkan, R., Hewitt, M., Dewey, M., Blair, M., Robinson, J., Williams, D. and Brummell, K. (2000) 'Does home visiting improve parenting and the quality of the home environment? A systematic review and meta analysis', *Archive of Disease in Childhood*, 82: 443–451.

Kennedy, B. P., Kawachi, I. and Kennedy, B. P. (1998) 'Mortality, the social environment, crime and violence', *Sociology of Health and Illness*, 20: 578–597.

Kessler, R., Berglund, P., Demler, O., Jin, R., Merikangas, K.R., and Walters, E.E. (2005) 'Lifetime prevalence and age-of-onset distributions of DSM-IV disorders in the National Comorbidity Survey Replication', *Archives of General Psychiatry*, 62(6): 593.

Keyes, C.M. (1998) 'Social well-being', *Social Psychology Quarterly*, 61: 121–40.

Keyes, C. (2006) 'Subjective well-being in mental health and human development research worldwide: an introduction', *Social Indicators Research*, 77(1): 1–10.

Keyes, C. L. (2007) 'Promoting and protecting mental health as flourishing: a complementary strategy for improving national mental health', *Am Psychol.*, 62(2): 95–108.

Keyes, C. (2010) *Flourishing*. Available from *Corsini Encyclopedia of Psychology*. (accessed 15 January 2013).

Keyes, C., Shmotkin, D. and Ryff, C. (2002) 'Optimizing well-being: the empirical encounter of two traditions', *Journal of Personality and Social Psychology*, 82(6): 1007–1022.

Keyes, C. L. M. and Annas, J. (2009) 'Feeling good and functioning well: distinctive concepts in ancient philosophy and contemporary science', *The Journal of Positive Psychology*, 4: 197–201.

Kidger, J., Donovan, J. L., Biddle, L., Campbell, R. and Gunnell, D. (2009) 'Supporting adolescent emotional health in schools: a mixed methods study of student and staff views in England', *BMC Public Health*, 9: 403.

Kim-Cohen, J., Caspi, A., Moffitt, T. E., Milne, B. J. and Poulton, R. (2003) 'Prior juvenile diagnoses in adults with mental disorder – Developmental follow-back of a prospective longitudinal cohort', *Archives of General Psychiatry*, 60: 709–717.

Kleinman, A. (1987) 'Anthropology and psychiatry: the role of culture in cross-cultural research on illness', *British Journal of Psychiatry*, 151: 447–454.

Kloppenburg, R. P., van den Berg, E., Kappelle, L. J. and Biessels, G. J. (2008) 'Diabetes and other vascular risk factors for dementia: which factor matters most? A systematic review', *European Journal of Pharmacology*, 585: 97–108.

Knapp, M., Bauer, A., Perkins, M. and Snell, T. (2010) *Building Community Capacity: Making an Economic Case*. London: PSSRU Discussion Paper 2772. www.pssru.ac.uk/pdf/dp2772.pdf (accessed 25 March 2013).

Knapp, M., McDaid, D. and Parsonage, M. (2011) *Mental Health Promotion and Mental Illness Prevention: The Economic Case*. London: Department of Health.

Knapp, M. (PSSRU, London School of Economics) and McCrone, P. (King's College London, Institute of Psychiatry) (2011) speaking at a conference on Best Practice in Mental Health GP-led Commissioning, Cambridge, 25 March.

Knol M.J., Twisk J.W., Beekman A.T., Heine R.J., Snoek F.J. and Pouwer F. (2006) 'Depression as a risk factor for the onset of type 2 diabetes mellitus: A meta-analysis', *Diabetologia*, 49(5):837–45.

Konow, J. and Early, J. (2008) 'The hedonistic paradox: is homo economicus happier?', *Journal of Public Economics*, 92: 1–33.

Kretzmann, J. P. and McKnight, J. L. (1993) *Building Communities from the Inside Out: A Path Toward Finding and Mobilizing a Community's Assets*. Evanston, IL: Institute for Policy Research.

Kubzansky, L.D. and Thurston, R.C. (2007) 'Emotional Vitality and Incident Coronary Heart Disease: Benefits of Healthy Psychological Functioning', *Arch Gen Psychiatry.*, 64(12): 1393–1401.

Kuh, D. and Ben-Shlomo, Y. (1997) *A Life Course Approach to Chronic Disease Epidemiology*. Oxford: Oxford University Press.

Kuhlman, K. R., Howell, K. H. G. and Graham-Bermann, S. A. (2012) 'Physical health in preschool children exposed to intimate partner violence', *Journal of Family Violence*, 27: 499–510.

Lampinen, P., Heikkinen, R. L., Kauppinen, M. and Heikkinen, E. (2006) 'Activity as a predictor of mental wellbeing among older adults', *Aging and Mental Health*, 10 (5): 454–466.

Lee, S., Altschul, I. and Mowbray, C. (2008) 'Using planned adaptation to implement evidence-based programmes with new populations', *American Journal of Community Psychology*, 41: 290–303.

Leventhal, T. and Brooks-Gunn, J. (2000) 'The neighborhoods they live in: the effects of neighborhood residence upon child and adolescent outcomes', *Psychological Bulletin*, 126(309): 337.

Lewin, J. (2010) 'Perinatal psychiatric disorders', in D. Kohen (ed.) *Oxford Textbook of Women and Mental Health*. Oxford: Oxford University Press, pp. 161–168.

Lindsay, G., Strand, S., Davis, H., Band, S., Cullen, M. A., Cullen, S., Hasluck, C., Evans, R. and Stewart-Brown, S. (2008) *Parenting Early Intervention Pathfinder Evaluation*. London: Department for Children, Schools and Families.

Lister-Sharp, D., Chapman, S., Stewart-Brown, S. and Sowden, A. (1999) 'Health promoting schools and health promotion in schools: two systematic reviews', *Health Technology Assessment*, 3(22).

Liu, X., Tein, J. Y., Sandler, I. N. and Zhao, Z. (2005) 'Psychopathology associated with suicide attempts among rural adolescents of China', *Suicide and Life-Threatening Behavior*, 35(3): 265–276.

Liu, X., Tein, J. Y. and Zhao, Z. (2004) 'Coping strategies and behavioral/emotional problems among Chinese adolescents', *Psychiatry Research*, 126(3): 275–285.

Lobato, G., Moraes, C. L., Dias, A. S. and Reichenheim, M. E. (2012) 'Alcohol misuse among partners: a potential effect modifier in the relationship between physical intimate partner violence and postpartum depression', *Social Psychiatry and Psychiatric Epidemiology*, 47: 427–438.

Lorenc, T., Clayton, S., Neary, D., Whitehead, M., Petticrew, M., Thomson, H., Cummins, S., Sowden, A. and Renton, A. (2012) 'Crime, fear of crime, environment and mental health and wellbeing: mapping review of theories and causal pathways', *Health and Place*, 18: 757–765.

Lowery, J., Aron, D., Keith, R., Kirsch, S. and Alexander, J. (2009) 'Fostering implementation of health services research findings into practice: a consolidated framework for advancing implementation science'. Biomed.Open access.

Lu, L. and Shih, J. B. (1997) 'Sources of happiness: a qualitative approach', *Journal of Social Psychology*, 137(2): 181–197.

Lu, M.C. and Halfon, N. (2003) 'Racial and ethnic disparities in birth outcomes: a life-course perspective', *Matern Child Health J.*,7(1):13–30.

Lucas, R. E. (2007) 'Long-term disability is associated with lasting changes in subjective well-being: evidence from two nationally representative longitudinal studies', *Journal of Personality and Social Psychology*, 92(4): 717–730.

Luchsinger, J. A. (2010) 'Diabetes, related conditions, and dementia', *Journal of the Neurological Sciences*, 299(1): 35–38.

Lyon, A. and Halliday, M. (2005) *'It wisnae me': Climate Change and Mental Health in the 21st Century*. St Andrews, Scotland: International Futures Forum.

Lyubomirsky, S., Sheldon, K. M. and Schkade, D. (2005) 'Pursuing happiness: the architecture of sustainable change', *Review of General Psychology*, 9: 111–131.

Maggi, S., Roberts, W., MacLennan, D. and D'Sngiull, A. (2011) 'Community resilience, quality childcare, and preschoolers' mental health: a three-city comparison', *Social Science and Medicine*, 73(7): 1080–1087.

Manthorpe, J. and Illife, S. (2011) 'Social work with older people-reducing suicide risk: a critical review of practice and prevention', *British Journal of Social Work*, 41(1): 131–147.

Marmot, M. (2010) *Fair Society, Healthy Lives: A Strategic Review of Health Inequalities in England Post-2010 (The Marmot Review)*. London: University College London.

Maslow, A. H. (1943) 'A theory of human motivation', *Psychological Review*, 50(4): 370–396.

May, C. (2006) 'A rational model for assessing and evaluating complex interventions in health care', *BMC Health Services Research*, 6(1): 86.

McAuley, E., Motl, R. W., Morris, K. S., Hu, L., Doerksen, S. E., Elavsky, S. and Konopack, J. F. (2007) 'Enhancing physical activity adherence and well-being in multiple sclerosis: a randomised controlled trial', *Multiple Sclerosis Journal*, 13(5): 652–659.

McCrone, P., Dhanasiri, S., Patel, A., Knapp, M. and Lawton-Smith, S. (2008) *Paying the Price: The Cost of Mental Health Care in England to 2026*. London: King's Fund.

McDaid, D. and Park, A.-L. (2011) 'Investing in mental health and well-being: findings from the DataPrev project', *Health Promotion International*, 26(S1): i108–i139.

McDaniel, B., Braiden, H. J. and Regan, H. (2010) *The Incredible Years Parenting Programme: Believe in Children*. Belfast: Northern Ireland Barnardos.

McLean, J. (2011) *Asset Based Approaches for Health Improvement: Redressing the Balance*. Glasgow: Glasgow Centre for Population Health.

Meade, C. and Lamb, P. (2007) *Family Learning Matters Topic Paper 3. Family Learning to Employment: Raising Aspirations and Gaining Skills*. London: NIACE.

Meier, A. (2002) 'An online stress management support group for social workers', *Journal of Technology in Human Services* 20 (1–2): 107–132.

Meltzer, H., Gatward, R., Corbin, T., Goodman, R. and Ford, T. (2003) *Persistence, Onset, Risk Factors and Outcomes of Childhood Mental Disorders*. London: The Stationery Office.

Menon, R. and Farina, C. (2011) 'Shared Molecular and Functional Frameworks among Five Complex Human Disorders: A Comparative Study on Interactomes Linked to Susceptibility Genes', *PLoS ONE* 6(4): e18660.

Messer, L., Kaufman, J., Dole, N., Herring, A. and Laraia, B. (2006) 'Violent crime exposure classification and adverse birth outcomes: a geographically-defined cohort study', *International Journal of Health Geographics*, 5: 22.

Meyer, J. H. F. and Land, R. (2003) 'Threshold concepts and troublesome knowledge: linkages to ways of thinking and practising within the disciplines', in C. Rust (ed.), *Improving Student Learning: Improving Student Learning Theory and Practice – Ten Years On*. Oxford: Oxford Centre for Staff and Learning Development.

Meyer, J. H. F. and Land, R. (2005) 'Threshold concepts and troublesome knowledge (2): epistemological considerations and a conceptual framework for teaching and learning', *Higher Education*, 49, 373–388.

Mezuk, B., Eaton, W. W., Albrecht, S. and Golden, S. H. (2008) 'Depression and type 2 diabetes over the lifespan', *Diabetes Care*, 31: 2383–2390.

Michie, S. and Williams, S. (2003) 'Reducing work related psychological ill health and sickness absence: a systematic literature review', *Occupational and Environmental Medicine*, 60: 3–9.

Mihalic, S. (2002) *The Importance of Implementation Fidelity*, http://incredibleyears.comwww.incredibleyears.com/Library/items/fidelity-importance.pdf (accessed 25 March 2013).

Milgrom, J., Schembri, C., Ericksen, J., Ross, J. and Gemmill, A. W. (2011) 'Towards parenthood: an antenatal intervention to reduce depression, anxiety and parenting difficulties', *Journal of Affective Disorders*, 130: 385–394.

Miller, G. E., Chen, E. and Parker, K. J. (2011a) 'Psychological stress in childhood and susceptibility to the chronic diseases of aging: moving toward a model of behavioral and biological mechanisms', *Psychological Bulletin*, 137(6): 959–997.

Miller, G.E., Lachman, M.E., Chen, E., Gruenewald, T.L., Karlamangla, A.S. and Seeman, T.E. (2011b) 'Pathways to Resilience', *Psychological Science*, 22(12): 1591–1599.

Miller, I. J. and Ruckstalis, M. (1999) 'Hypotheses about post-partum reactivity', in L. J. Miller (ed.), *Postpartum Mood Disorder*. Washington DC: American Psychiatric Press, pp. 262–265.

Miller, S., Lo, C., Gagliese, L., Hales, S., Rydall, A., Zimmermann, C., Li, M. and Rodin, G. (2011c) 'Patterns of depression in cancer patients: an indirect test of gender-specifc vulnerabilities to depression', *Social Psychiatry and Psychiatric Epidemiology*, 46(8): 767–774.

Mills, P. R., Kessler, R. C., Cooper, J. and Sullivan, S. (2007) 'Impact of a health promotion program on employee health risks and work productivity', *American Journal of Health Promotion*, 22(1): 45–53.

Milton, B., Moonan, M., Taylor-Robinson, D., and Whitehead, M. (eds) (2011) How can the health equity impact of universal policies be evaluated? Insights into approaches and next steps. Synthesis of discussions from an expert group meeting. Liverpool, November 2-4, 2010. World Health Organization. Retrieved from: www.euro.who.int/__data/assets/pdf_file/0019/155062/E95912.pdf

Mimura, C. and Griffiths, P. (2003) 'The effectiveness of current approaches to workplace stress management in the nursing profession: an evidence based literature review', *Occupational and Environmental Medicine*, 60: 10–15.

Misri, S., Kostaras, X., Fox, D. and Kostaras, D. (2000) 'The impact of partner support in the treatment of postpartum depression', *Canadian Journal of Psychiatry*, 45(6): 554–558.

Mooney, G. H. (1983) 'Equity in health care: confronting the confusion', *Effectiveness in Health Care*, 1(4): 179–185.

Mordacci, R. S. and Sobel, R. (1998) 'Health: a comprehensive concept', *Journal of Medical Internet Research*, 28(1): 34–38.

Morrell, C. J., Warner, R., Slade, P., Dixon, S., Walters, S., Paley, G. and Brugha, T. (2009) 'Psychological interventions for postnatal depression: cluster randomised trial and economic evaluation. The PoNDER trial', *Health Technology Assessment*, 13(30).

Mottusa, R., Galea, C. R., Starra, J. M. and Dearya, I. J. (2012) '"On the street where you live": Neighbourhood deprivation and quality of life among community-dwelling older people in Edinburgh, Scotland', *Social Science and Medicine*, 74(9): 1368–1374.

Mozaffarian, D., Kamineni, A., Carnethon, M., Djoussé, L., Ukamal, K. J. and Iscovick, D. (2009) 'Lifestyle risk factors and new-onset diabetes mellitus in older adults: the cardiovascular health study', *Archives of Internal Medicine*. 169(8): 798–807.

MSD (2013) *Implementing the NICE Quality Standard for Diabetes as Part of the NHS Outcomes Framework*. MSD.

MS Society Blog (27 September 2012). David Rowland Alice Hamilton

Murray, L., Arteche, A., Fearon, P., Halligan, S., Croudace, T. and Cooper, P. (2010) 'The effects of maternal postnatal depression and child sex on academic performance at age 16 years: a developmental approach', *Journal of Child Psychology and Psychiatry*, 51(10): 1150–1159.

Murray, L., Arteche, A., Fearon, P., Halligan, S., Goodyer, I. and Cooper, P. (2011) 'Maternal postnatal depression and the development of depression in offspring up to 16 years of age', *Journal of the American Academy of Child and Adolescent Psychiatry*, 50(5): 460–470.

Murray, L. and Cooper, P. J. (2003) 'Intergenerational transmission of affective and cognitive processes associated with depression: infancy and the pre-school years', in I. M. Goodyer (ed.), *Unipolar Depression: A Lifespan Perspective.* Oxford: Oxford University Press, pp. 17–46.

Murray, L., Fiori-Cowley, A., Hooper, R. and Cooper, P. (1996a) 'The impact of postnatal depression and associated adversity on early mother-infant interactions and later infant outcome', *Child Development,* 67: 2512–2526.

Murray, L., Hipwell, R., Stein, A. and Cooper, P. (1996b) 'The cognitive development of 5-year-old children of postnatally depressed mothers', *Journal of Child Psychology and Psychiatry,* 37: 927–935.

Murray, L., Sinclair, D., Cooper, P., Ducournau, P., Turner, P. and Stein, A. (1999) 'The socioemotional development of 5-year-old children of postnatally depressed mothers', *Journal of Child Psychology and Psychiatry,* 40(8): 1259–1271.

Myerson, L. A., Long, R. M. Jr. and Marx, B. P. (2002) 'The influence of childhood sexual abuse, physical abuse, family environment, and gender on the psychological adjustment of adolescents', *Child Abuse and Neglect,* 26(4): 387–405.

Nabi, H., Kivimaki, M., Suominen, S., Koskenvuo, M., Singh-Manooux, A. and Vahtera, J. (2010) 'Does depression predict coronary heart disease and cerebrovascular disease equally well? The Health and Social Support Prospective Cohort Study', *International Journal of Epidemiology,* 39(4): 1016–1024.

Narayan, K. M. V., Echouffo-Tcheugui, J. B., Mohan, V. and Ali, M. K. (2012) 'Global prevention and control of type 2 diabetes will require paradigm shifts in policies within and among countries', *Health Affairs,* 31(1): 84–92.

National Collaborating Centre for Methods and Tools (2009). *Tool for Grading Public Health Interventions* (NICE Tool). Hamilton, ON: McMaster University.

National Mental Wellbeing Impact Assessment (MWIA) Collaborative (2011). *Mental Well-being Impact Assessment: A Tooolkit for Well-being.* London: National MWIA Collaborative (England).

nef (New Economics Foundation) (2002)*The Time Of Our Lives: Using time banking for neighbourhood renewal and community capacity building.* London: nef.

nef (New Economics Foundation) (2012) *Well-being patterns uncovered: An analysis of UK data.* London: nef.

Nesta (2012) *People Powered Health Co-production Catalogue,* www.nesta.org.uk/library/documents/PPH_v13.pdf (accessed 20 March 2013).

Newbigging, K., Bola, M. and Shah, A. (2008) *Scoping Exercise with Black and Minority Ethnic Groups on Perceptions of Mental Wellbeing in Scotland.* Glasgow: NHS Scotland.

Newbigging, K. and Heginbotham, C. (2010) *Commissioning Mental Wellbeing for All: A Toolkit for Commissioners.* Preston: University of Central Lancashire. www.nmhdu.org.uk/silo/files/commissioning-wellbeing-for-all.pdf.

NHS Confederation (2012a) *Patient and Public Engagement for Health and Wellbeing Boards: A Review of Resources,* www.nhsconfed.org/Publications/Documents/Patient_and_public_engagement_health_wellbeing_boards210612.pdf (accessed 10 March 2013).

NHS Confederation (2012b) *A Primary Care Approach to Mental Health and Wellbeing: Case Study Report on Sandwell.* London: NHS Confederation.

NHS Scotland (2010) *Towards a Mentally Flourishing Scotland: Policy and Action Plan Guidance to Support Local Implementation.* Online resource Available at: www.healthscotland.com/documents/4729.aspx (accessed 14 September 2013).

NICE (National Institute for Health and Clinical Excellence) (2006) Computerized cognitive behaviour therapy for depression and anxiety: Technology appraisal 97. London: National Institute for Clinical Excellence.

NICE (National Institute for Health and Clinical Excellence) (2007a) Antenatal and postnatal mental health: Clinical management and service management. NICE clinical guideline 45. Anxiety (amended). London: National Institute for Clinical Excellence.

NICE (National Institute for Health and Clinical Excellence) (2007b) Depression: management of depression in primary and secondary care. NICE clinical guideline 23 (amended). London: National Institute for Clinical Excellence.

NICE (National Institute for Health and Clinical Excellence) (2008a) *Mental Wellbeing and Older People* (PH 16). *Occupational Therapy Interventions and Physical Activity Interventions to Promote the Mental Wellbeing of Older People in Primary Care and Residential Care*. London: NICE.

NICE (National Institute for Health and Clinical Excellence) (2008b) *Promoting and Creating Built or Natural Environments that Encourage and Support Physical Activity*. London: NICE.

NICE (National Institute for Health and Clinical Excellence) (2008c) An assessment of community engagement and community development approaches including the collaborative methodology and community champions. Public health guidance, PH9.

NICE (National Institute for Health and Clinical Excellence) (2009a) *Depression in Adults (Update)* (CG90). London: NICE.

NICE (National Institute for Health and Clinical Excellence) (2009b) *Depression in Adults with a Chronic Physical Health Problem: Treatment and Management* (CG91). London: NICE.

NICE (National Institute for Health and Clinical Excellence) (2010) *Alcohol Use Disorders: Preventing Harmful Drinking* (PH24). London: NICE.

NICE (National Institute for Health and Clinical Excellence) (2011) *Quality Standards Programme. Quality Standards for Diabetes in Adults* (QS6). London: NICE.

North Yorkshire County Council (2007) *Strategic Commissioning for Independence, Well-being and Choice: Strategic Commissioning for Adult Social Care in North Yorkshire for the Next 15 Years, 2007–2022*. North Yorkshire County Council Adult and Community Services.

O'Connor, T. G., Heron, J., Glover, V. and Alspac Study Team (2002) 'Antenatal anxiety predicts child behavioral/emotional problems independently of postnatal depression', *Journal of the American Academy of Child and Adolescent Psychiatry*, 41(12): 1470–1477.

Oddy, W. H., Kendall, G. E., Li, J., Jacoby, P., Robinson, M., de Klerk, N. H., Silburn, S. R., Zubrick, S. R., Landau, L. I. and Stanley, F. J. (2010) 'The long-term effects of breastfeeding on child and adolescent mental health: a pregnancy cohort study followed for 14 years', *The Journal of Pediatrics*, 156(4): 568–574.

Okun, M. A., Stock, W. A., Haring, M. J. and Witter, R. A. (1984) 'Health and subjective well-being: a meta-analysis', *The International Journal of Ageing and Human Development*, 19(2): 111–132.

Olafsdottir, A. E., Reidpath, D. E., Pokhrel, S. and Allotey, P. (2011) 'Health systems performance in sub-Saharan Africa: governance, outcome and equity', *BMC Public Health*, 11: 237.

The Older People's Health and Wellbeing Atlas accessed online at www.wmpho.org.uk/olderpeopleatlas/data.aspx, which is now part of Public Health England.

Olds, D. L. (2002) 'Prenatal and home visiting by nurses: from randomised control trials to community replication', *Prevention Science* (official journal of the Society for Prevention Research), 3(3): 153–172.

Olds, D., Henderson, C.R., Cole, R., Eckenrode, J., Kitzman, H., Luckey, D., Pettitt, L., Sidora, K., Morris, P. and Powers, J. (1998) 'Long-term effects of nurse home visitation on children's criminal and antisocial behavior – 15-year follow-up of a randomized controlled trial', *Journal of The American Medical Association*, 280(14): 1238–1244.

ONS (Office for National Statistics) (2010) *Measuring National Well-being: Consultation Document*.

Onyike, C. U., Crum, R.M., Lee, H.B., Lyketsos, C.G. and Eaton, W.W. (2003) 'Is Obesity Associated with Major Depression? Results from the Third National Health and Examination Survey', *American Journal of Epidemiology*, 158 (12): 1139–1147.

Osborn, D. P., Levy, G., Nazareth, I., Petersen, I., Islam, A. and King, M. B. (2007) 'Relative risk of cardiovascular and cancer mortality in people with severe mental illness from the United Kingdom's General Practice Research Database', *Archives of General Psychiatry*, 64(2): 242–249.

Östlin, P., Schrecker, T., Sadana, R., Bonnefoy, J., Gilson, L., Hertzman, C. and et al. (2011) 'Priorities for research on equity and health: towards an equity-focused health research agenda', *PLoS Med*, 8 (11). www.plosmedicine.org/article/info%3Adoi%2F10.1371%2Fjournal.pmed.1001115 (accessed 7 March 2013).

Owen, L., Morgan, A., Fischer, A., Ellis, S., Hoy, A. and Kelly, M. P. (2012) 'The cost-effectiveness of public health interventions', *Journal of Public Health*, 34: 37–45.

Parkinson, J. (2007) *Review of Scales of Positive Mental Health Validated for Use with Adults in the UK: Technical Report*. Edinburgh: Health Scotland.

Pavlekovic, G., Pluemer, K. D., Vaandrager, L., et al. (2011) *Twenty Years of Capacity Building. Evolution of Salutogenic Training: The ETC 'Healthy Learning' Process*. Zagreb: European Training Consortium in Public Health and Health Promotion (ETC-PHHP and the Andrija Stampar School of Public Health).

Payton, J., Wessberg, R. P., Durlak, J. A., Dymnicki, A.B., Taylor, R.D. Schellinger, K.B. and Pachan, M. (2008) *The Positive Impact of Social and Emotional Learning for Kindergarten to Eighth Grade Students: Findings from Three Scientific Reviews*. Chicago, IL: Collaborative for Academic, Social and Emotional Learning.

Penedo, F. J. and Dahn, J. R. (2005) 'Exercise and well-being: a review of mental and physical health benefits associated with physical activity', *Current Opinion in Psychiatry*, 18(2): 189–193.

Perk, J. and European Association for Cardiovascular Prevention and Rehabilitation (2012) 'European Guidelines on cardiovascular disease prevention in clinical practice', *European Heart Journal*, 3(1635): 1635–1701.

Petrie, J., Bunn, F. and Byrne, G. (2007) 'Parenting programmes for preventing tobacco, alcohol and drug misuse in children <18 years: a systematic review', *Health Education Research*, 22: 177–191.

Pickin, C., Popay, J., Staely, K., Bruce, N. and Jones, C. (2002) 'Developing a model to enhance the capacity of statutory organisations to engage with lay communities', *Journal of Health Services Research and Policy*, 7(1).

Pies, C., Parthasarathy, P. and Posner, S. F. (2012) 'Integrating the life course perspective into a local maternal and child health program', *Journal of Maternal and Child Health*, 16: 649–655.

Poobalan, A. S., Aucott, L. S., Ross, L., Smith, W. C. S., Helms, P. J. and Williams, J. H. (2007) 'Effects of treating postnatal depression on mother-infant interaction and child development: systematic review', *British Journal of Psychiatry*, 191: 378–386.

Popay, J. (2006) Community Engagement, community development and health improvement. A Background Paper prepared for NICE.

Popay, J. (2012) Informal communication, *In Global Health Equity in Times of Crisis*, symposium, 31 October 2012, E. Missoni (coordinator), Geneva: GHEF.

Popay, J., Attree, P., Hornby, D.,Milton, B., Whitehead, M., French, B., Kowarzik, U., Simpson, N., Povall, S. (2007) *Community Engagement in Initiatives Addressing the Wider Social Determinants of Health: A Rapid Review of Evidence on Impact, Experience and Process*. Lancaster: Universities of Lancaster, Liverpool and Central Lancashire.

Power, A. K. (2010) 'Transforming the nation's health: next steps in mental health promotion', *American Journal of Public Health*, 100: 2343–2346.

Purshouse, R., Brennan, A., Latimer, N., Meng, Y., Rafia, R., Jackson, R. and Meier, P. (2009) *Public Health Related Strategies and Interventions to Reduce Alcohol Attributable Harm in England Using the Sheffield Alcohol Policy Model Version 2.0. Report to the NICE Public Health Programme Development Group*, Sheffield: University of Sheffield.

RCPsych (2010) *No Health Without Public Mental Health*. London: Royal College of Psychiatrists.

Reaveley, N., Livingston, J., Buchbinder, R., Bennell, K., Stecki, C. and Osborne, R.H. (2010) 'A systematic grounded approach to the development of complex interventions: The Australian WorkHealth Program – Arthritis as a case study', *Soc. Sci. Med.*, 70 (3): 342–350.

Reed, S. (2001) http://cllrstevereed.wordpress.com/2011/07/15/coopcouncils/ (accessed on 18/04/2013).

Renn, B. N., Feliciano, L. and Segal, D. L. (2011) 'The bidirectional relationship of depression and diabetes: a systematic review', *Clinical Psychology Review*, 31: 1239–1246.

Reynolds, A. J., J. A. Temple, D. L. Robertson, and Mann, E. A. (2001) 'Long-term effects of an early childhood intervention on educational achievement and juvenile arrest: A 15-year follow-up of low-income children in public schools', *JAMA* 285: 2339–2346.

Robinson, D. and Horwitz, W. (2012) *Shifting to Prevention: Overcoming the Structural Barriers.* London: New Economics Foundation.

Rozanski, A., Blumenthal, J.A., Davidson, K.W., Saab P.G. And Kubzansky, L. (2005) 'The epidemiology, pathophysiology, and management of psychosocial risk factors in cardiac practice: the emerging field of behavioral cardiology', *J Am Coll Cardiol.* 45(5):637–51.

Rushey Green Timebank (2009) Available at www.cihm.leeds.ac.uk/new/wp-content/uploads/2009/05/Rushey-Green-Time-Bank.pdf

Russell, D., Springer, K. W. and Greefield, E. A. (2010) 'Witnessing domestic abuse in childhood as an independent risk factor for depressive symptoms in young adulthood', *Child Abuse and Neglect,* 34(6): 448–453.

Rustad, J. K., Musselman, D. L. and Nemeroff, C. B. (2011) 'The relationship of depression and diabetes: pathophysiological and treatment implications', *Psychoneuroendocrinology,* 36: 1276–1286.

Ryan, R. M. and Deci, E. L. (2001) 'On happiness and human potentials: a review of research on hedonic and eudaimonic well-being', *Annual Review of Psychology,* 52: 141–166.

Rychetnik, L., Frommer, M., Hawe, P. and Shiell, A. (2002) 'Criteria for evaluating evidence on public health interventions', *Journal of Epidemiology and Community Health,* 56: 119–127.

Sanders, M. (1999) 'The Triple P – Positive Parenting Program: towards an empirically validated multilevel parenting and family support strategy for the prevention of behavior and emotional problems in children', *Clinical Child and Family Psychology Review,* 2: 71–90.

Saxena, S., Jane-Llopis, E. and Hosmans, C. (2006) 'Prevention of mental and behavioural disorders: implications for policy and practice', *World Psychiatry,* 5(1): 5–14.

Schachter, H. M., Girardi, A., Ly, M., Lacroix, D., Lumb, A. B., van Berkom, J. and Gill, R. (2008) 'Effects of school-based interventions on mental health stigmatisation: a systematic review', *Child and Adolescent Psychiatry and Mental Health,* 2(1): 18.

Scharloo, M., Kaptein, A. and Weinman, J. (2000) 'Physical and psychological correlates of functioning in patients with chronic obstructive pulmonary disease', *Journal of Asthma,* 37: 17–29.

Scott, S., Knapp, M., Henderson, J. and Maughan, B. (2001a) 'Financial cost of social exclusion: follow up study of antisocial children into adulthood', *British Medical Journal,* 323: 191.

Scott, S., O'Connor, T. G. and Futh, A. (2006) *What Makes Parenting Programmes Work in Disadvantaged Areas? The PALS Trial.* York: Joseph Rowntree Foundation, www.jrf.org.uk/publications/what-makes-parenting-programmes-work-disadvantaged-areas (accessed 18 August 2012).

Scott, S., O'Connor, T., Futh, A., Price, J., Matias, C. and Doolan, M. (2010) 'Impact of a parenting program in a high-risk, multi-ethnic community: The PALS trial', *Journal of Child, Psychology and Psychiatry,* 51: 1331–1341.

Scott, S., Spender, Q., Doolan, M., Jacobs, B. and Asplan, H. (2001b) 'Multicentre controlled trial of parenting groups for childhood antisocial behaviour in clinical practice', *British Medical Journal,* 323: 194.

Secretary of State for Health (2010) *Healthy Lives, Healthy People: Our strategy for Public Health in England.* Cmnd 7985. London: HM Government.

Secretary of State for Health (2012) *The Government's Alcohol Strategy.* Cm 8336. London: Department of Health.

Secretary of State for Health (2013) *Healthy Lives, Healthy People: Update and Way Forward.* Cm 8134. London: The Stationery Office.

Sen, A. (2002) 'Why health equity?', *Health Economics,* 11(8): 659–666.

Seymour, L. and Grove, B. (2005) *Workplace Interventions for People with Common Mental Health Problems.* London: British Occupational Health Research Foundation, www.bohrf.org.uk/downloads/cmh_rev.pdf (accessed 20 March 2013).

Sharpley, M.S., Hutchinson, G., Murray, R.M. and McKenzie, K. (2001) 'Understanding the excess of psychosis among the African—Caribbean population in England: Review of current hypotheses', *B. J. Psychiatry,* 178: s60–s68.

Simkiss, D. E., Snooks, H. A., Stallard, N., Davies, S., Thomas, M. A., Anthony, B., Winstanley, S., Wilson, L. and Stewart-Brown, S. (2010) 'Measuring the impact and costs of a universal group based parenting programme: protocol and implementation of a trial', *BMC Public Health*, 10: 364.

Simon, G. E., Katon, W. J., Lin, E. H. B., Rutter, C., Manning, W. G., Von Korff, M., Ciechanowski, P., Ludman, E. J. and Young, B. A. (2007) 'Cost-effectiveness of systematic depression treatment among people with diabetes mellitus', *Archives of General Psychiatry*, 64(1): 65–72.

Small, M. L. (2009) *Unanticipated Gains: Origins of Network Inequality in Everyday Life*. New York: Oxford University Press.

Smith, L. F. and Corlett, S. K. (2011) 'The Lambeth Wellbeing and Happiness Programme: a strategic approach to public mental health', *Social Work and Social Sciences Review*, 14(3): 23–36.

Solar, O. and Irwin, A. (2007) *A Conceptual Framework for Action on the Social Determinants of Health*. WHO Commission on the Social Determinants of Health.

Stead, M., Gordon, R., Angus, K., and McDermott, L. (2007) 'A systematic review of social marketing effectiveness'. *Health Education*, 107(2): 126–191.

Steel, P., Schmidt, J. and Shultz, J. (2008) 'Refining the relationship between personality and subjective well-being', *Psychological Bulletin*, 134(1): 138–161.

Stegeman, I. and Costongs, C. (eds) (2012) *The Right Start to a Healthy Life*. Brussels: EuroHealthNet.

Steger, M. F. and Kashdan, T. B. (2009) 'Depression and everyday social activity, belonging, and wellbeing', *Journal of Counseling Psychology*, 56(2): 289–300.

Stern, N. (2006) *The Economics of Climate Change: The Stern Review*. Cambridge: Cambridge University Press.

Stevahn, L., Johnson, D., Johnson, R., Schultz, R. (2002) 'Effects of Conflict Resolution Training Integrated Into a High School Social Studies Curriculum', *Journal of Social Psychology*, 142(3): 305–331.

Stewart, R. and Brownlow, J. (1985) *Myself: A Descriptive Report*. Newcastle, UK: Northern Mind.

Stuckler, D., Basu, S., Suhrcke, M., Coutts, A., and McKee, M. (2009). 'The public health effect of economic crises and alternative policy responses in Europe: an empirical analysis', *The Lancet*, 374(9686): 315–323.

Suhonen, R., Stolt, M., Puro, M. and Leino-Kilpi, H. (2011) 'Individuality in older people's care – challenges for the development of nursing and nursing management', *Journal of Nursing Management*, 19(7): 883–896.

Sundquist, K., Theobald, H., Yang, M., Li, X., Johansson, S. E. and Sundquist, J. (2006) 'Neighborhood violent crime and unemployment increase the risk of coronary heart disease: a multilevel study in an urban setting', *Social Science and Medicine*, 62: 2061–2071.

Surtees, P. G., Wainwright, N. W. J., Luben, R. N., Wareham, N. J., Bingham, S. A. and Khaw, K. T. (2008) 'Psychological distress, major depressive disorder and risk of stroke', *Neurology*, 70(788): 794.

Svetaz, V., Ireland, M. and Blum, R. (2000) 'Adolescents with learning disabilities: risk and protective factors associated with emotional well being: findings from the national longitudinal study of adolescent health', *Journal of Adolescent Health*, 27: 340–348.

Sznitman, S.R., Reisel, L., Romer, D. (2011) 'The Neglected Role of Adolescent Emotional Well-Being in National Educational Achievement: Bridging the Gap Between Education and Mental Health Policies', *Journal of Adolescent Health*, 48, (2): 135–142.

Tadros, G. (2011) *Rapid Assessment Interface Discharge (RAID)*. Birmingham: Birmingham and Solihull Mental Health NHS Foundation Trust.

Taft, A. J., Small, R., Hegarty, K. L., Lumley, J., Watson, L. F. and Gold, L. (2009) 'MOSAIC (MOthers' Advocates In the Community): protocol and sample description of a cluster randomised trial of mentor mother support to reduce intimate partner violence among pregnant or recent mothers', *BMC Public Health*, 9: 159.

Tameside and Glossop NHS, Tameside Strategic Partnership, and Derbyshire Dales and High Peak Local Strategic Partnership (2011) *Tameside and Glossop Mental Wellbeing Strategy 2011-2013*.

Tandon, S. D., Perry, D. F., Mendelson, T., Kemp, K. and Leis, J. A. (2011) 'Preventing perinatal depression in low-income home visiting clients: a randomized controlled trial', *Journal of Consulting and Clinical Psychology*, 79(5): 707–712.

Tay, L. and Diener, E. (2011) 'Needs and subjective well-being around the world', *Journal of Personality and Social Psychology*, 101(2): 336–354.

Taylor, C. A., Guterman, N. B., Shawna, L. J. and Rathouz, P. J. (2009) 'Intimate partner violence, maternal stress, nativity, and risk for maternal maltreatment of young children', *American Journal of Public Health*, 99(1): 175–183.

Tennant, R., Hiller, L., Fishwick, R., Platt, S., Joseph, S., Weich, S., Parkinson, J., Secker, J. and Stewart-Brown, S. L. (2007) 'The Warwick-Edinburgh Mental Well-being Scale (WEMWBS): development and UK validation', *Health and Quality of Life Outcomes*, 5(63): 1477–7525.

Thompson, M. P., Kingee, J. B. and Desai, S. (2004) 'Gender differences in long-term health consequences of physical abuse of children: data from a nationally representative survey', *American Journal of Public Health*, 94(4): 599–604.

Tiberius, V. and Plakias, A. (2010) 'Well-being', in J. Doris and Moral Psychology Research Group (eds), *The Moral Psychology Handbook*. Oxford: Oxford University Press.

Tidyman, M. (2004) *Making it Diverse: Mental Health Promotion and Black and Ethnic Minority Ethnic Groups*. London: Centre for Mental Health.

Tidyman, M., Gale, E., and Linda Seymour, L. (2004) *Celebrating our Cultures: Guidelines for Mental Health Promotion with Black and Minority Ethnic Communities*. London Department of Health.

Tomlinson, C. L., Patel, S., Meek, C., Herd, C. P., Clarke, C. E., Stowe, R., Shah, L., Sackley, C., Deane, K. H. O., Wheatley, K. and Ives, N. (2012) 'Physiotherapy intervention in Parkinson's disease: systematic review and meta-analysis', *British Medical Journal*, 345.

Tudor, K. (1996) *Mental Health Promotion: Paradigms and Practice*. London: Routledge.

Tuomilehto, J., Lindstrom, J., Eriksson, J. G., et al. (2001) 'Prevention of Type 2 diabetes mellitus by changes in lifestyle among subjects with impaired glucose tolerance', *New England Journal of Medicine*, 344(18): 1343–1350.

Turner, J. (2012) 'I made the decision in those moments to live or die – and chose to live', *The Times* (UK).

Turning Point (2011) *Project – Connected Care in Swindon*. www.turning-point.co.uk/community-commissioning/connected-care/projects/connected-care-in-swindon.aspx

UNICEF (2007) *Child Poverty in Perspective: An Overview of Child Well-being in Rich Countries. A Comprehensive Assessment of the Lives and Well-being of Children and Adolescents in the Economically Advanced Nations*, Innocenti Report Card No. 7. UNICEF, Innocenti Research Centre, Florence.

van den Berg, P., Neumark-Sztainer, D., Hannan, P. J. and Haines, J. (2007) 'Is Dieting Advice From Magazines Helpful or Harmful? Five-Year Associations With Weight-Control Behaviors and Psychological Outcomes in Adolescents', *Pediatrics*, 119 (1): e30–e37.

van der Klink, J. J., Blonk, R. W., Schene, A. H. and van Dijk, F. J. H. (2001) 'The benefits of interventions for work-related stress', *American Journal of Public Health*, 91: 270–276.

van der Klink, J. J., Blonk, R. W., Schene, A. H. and van Dijk, F. J. H. (2003) 'Reducing long term sickness absence by an activating intervention in adjustment disorders: a cluster randomised controlled design', *Occupational Environmental Medicine*, 60(429): 437.

Van Ootegem, L., Spillemaeckers, S. and . (2010) 'With a focus on well-being and capabilities', *The Journal of Socio-Economics*, 39(3): 384–390.

Velayudhan, L., Poppe, M., Archer, N., Proitsi, P., Brown, R. and Lovestone, S. (2010) 'Risk of developing dementia in people with diabetes and mild cognitive impairment', *British Journal of Psychiatry*, 196: 36–40.

Vuori, J. and Silvonen, J. (2005) 'The benefits of a preventive job search program on re-employment and mental health at two years follow up', *Journal of Occupational and Organisational Psychology*, 78: 43–52.

Walpole, S. C., Rasanathan, K. and Campbell-Lendrum, D. (2009) 'Natural and unnatural synergies: climate change policy and health equity', *Bulletin of the World Health Organization*, 87(10): 799–801.

Walters, G.D. (2000) 'Behavioral Self-Control Training for Problem Drinkers: A Meta-Analysis of Randomized Control Studies', *Behav Ther* 31: 135–149.

Warr, P. B. (1999) 'Wellbeing and the Workplace,' in D. Kahneman, E. Diener, and N. Schwarz (eds.), *Wellbeing: Foundations of Hedonic Psychology*, New York: Russell Sage Foundation.

Warr, P. B. (1987) *Work, Unemployment and Mental Health*. Oxford: Clarendon Press.

Webb, B. C., Simpson, S. L. and Hairston, K. G. (2011) 'From politics to parity: using a health disparities index to guide legislative efforts for health equity', *American Journal of Public Health*, 101(3): 554–560.

Webster-Stratton, C. (2006) *The Incredible Years*. Seattle: The Incredible Years.

Webster-Stratton, C. (2007) 'Tailoring The Incredible Years Parenting Program according to children's developmental needs and family risk factors', in J. Briesmeister and C. Schaefer (eds), *Handbook of Parent Training*. New Jersey: John Wiley and Sons.

Webster-Stratton, C. and Reid, M. J. (2009) 'The Incredible Years Program for children from infancy to pre-adolescence: prevention and treatment of behavior problems', in R. Murrihy, A. Kidman and T. Ollendick (eds), *Clinician's Handbook for the Assessment and Treatment of Conduct Problems in Youth*. New York: Springer Press.

Weich, S., Brugha, T. S., King, M. B., McManus, S., Bebbington, P., Jenkins, R., Cooper, C., McBride, O. and Stewart-Brown, S. L. (2011) 'Mental well-being and mental illness: findings from the Adult Psychiatric Morbidity Survey for England 2007', *The British Journal of Psychiatry*, 199(1): 23–28.

Weich, S. and Lewis, G. (1998) 'Poverty, unemployment and common mental disorders: a population based cohort study', *British Medical Journal*, 317: 115–119.

Weightman A, Ellis S, Cullum A, et al. (2005) *Grading Evidence and Recommendations for Public Health Interventions: Developing and Piloting a Framework*. London: Health Development Agency.

Weightman, A., Ellis, S., Sander, L. and Turley, R. (2013) *Grading Evidence and Recommendations for Public Health Interventions: Developing and Piloting a Framework*. London: Health Development Agency.

Welshman, J. (2007) *Policy, Poverty, and Parenting*. Bristol: The Policy Press.

Westerhof, G. J. and Keyes, C. L. M. (2010) 'Mental illness and mental health: the two continua model across the lifespan', *Journal of Adult Development*, 17(2): 110–119.

Whitehead, M. (1991) 'The concepts and principles of equity and health', *Health Promotion International*, 6(3): 217–228.

Whitehead, M., Popay, J. (2010) 'Swimming upstream? Taking action on the social determinants of health inequalities', *Social science & medicine*, 71(7):1234–6.

WHO (1978) Declaration of Alma Ata, at www.who.int/publications/almaata_declaration_en.pdf (accessed 16 April 2013).

WHO (World Health Organization) (2005) Urban Health Equity Assessment and Response Tool (Urban HEART). Kobe, Japan: World Health Organization Centre for Health Development, www.who.int/kobe_centre/measuring/urbanheart/en/ (accessed 11 March 2013).

WHO (World Health Organization) (2008) *Closing the Gap in a Generation: Health Equity through Action on the Social Determinants of Health. Commission on Social Determinants of Health: Final Report*. Geneva, Switzerland: World Health Organization.

Wiggins, M., Oakley, A.,Sawtell, M., Austerberry, H., Clemens, F., Elbourne, D. (2005a) *Teenage Parenthood and Social Exclusion: A multi-method study*. London: Social Science Research Report, Institute of Education, University of London

Wiggins, M., Rosato, M., Austerberry, H. Sawtell, M., Oliver, S. (2005b) *Sure Start Plus. National Evaluation: Final Report*. London: Social Science Research Report, Institute of Education, University of London

Wilding J. and Barton, M. (2007) *Evaluation of the Strengthening Families, Strengthening Communities Programme*. London: Race Equality Unit.

Wilding, J. and Barton, M. (2009). *Evaluation of the strengthening families, strengthening communities programme 2005/6 and 2006/7*. London: Race Equality Foundation.

Wilkinson, R.G., Kawachi, I., and Kennedy B (1998) 'Mortality, the social environment, crime and violence', *Sociology of Health and Illness,* 20:578–597.

Wilkinson, R. and Pickett, K. (2009) *The Spirit Level: Why More Equal Societies Almost Always Do Better.* London: Penguin Books.

William, W., Eaton, W.W., Haroutune Armenian, H., Joseph Gallo, J., Laurie Pratt, L., Daniel E. and Ford, D. E. (1996) 'Depression and Risk for Onset of Type II Diabetes: A prospective population-based study', *Diabetes Care*, 19 (10): 1097–1102.

Williams, F., Popay, J. and Oakley, A. (1999) *Welfare Research: A Critical Review.* London: UCL Press Ltd.

Windle, G., Hughes, D., Linck, P., Russell, I., Morgan, R., Woods, R., Burholt, V., Edwards, R. T., Reeves, C. and Yeo, S. T. (2008) *Public Health Interventions to Promote Mental Well-being in People Aged 65 and Over: Systematic Review of Effectiveness and Cost-effectiveness.* PHIAC 17.14 Mental Well-being and Older People: Review of Effectiveness and Cost. Institute of Medical and Social Care Research, University of Wales Bangor.

Wood, A. M., Froh, J. J. and Geraghty, A. W. A. (2010) 'Gratitude and well-being: A review and theoretical integration', *Clinical Psychology Review*, 30(7): 890–905.

Wood, A. M. and Tarrier, N. (2010) 'Positive clinical psychology: a new vision and strategy for integrated research and practice', *Clinical Psychology Review*, 30(7): 819–829.

Wright, A., McGorry, P., Harris, M., Jorm, A. and Pennel, K. (2006) 'Development and evaluation of a youth mental health community awareness campaign: the Compass Strategy', *BMC Public Health*, 6(1): 215.

Wu, S.-F. V., Huang, Y.-C., Liang, S.-Y., Wang, T.-J., Lee, M.-C. and Tung, H.-H. (2011) 'Relationships among depression, anxiety, self-care behaviour and diabetes education difficulties in patients with type-2 diabetes: a cross-sectional questionnaire survey', *International Journal of Nursing Studies*, 48: 1376–1383.

Wutzke, S. E., Conigrave, K. M., Saunders, J. B. and Hall, W. D. (2002)' The long-term effectiveness of brief interventions for unsafe alcohol consumption: a 10 year follow-up', *Addiction*, 97: 665–675.

Xu, W., Caracciolo, B., Winblad, B., Backman, L. and Qui, C. F. L. (2010) 'Accelerated progression from mild cognitive impairment to dementia in people with diabetes', *Diabetes*, 59(11): 2928.

Yelin, E., Mathias S.D., Buesching, D.P., Rowland, C., Calucin, R.Q., Fifer, S. (1996) 'The impact on unemployment of an intervention to increase recognition of previously untreated anxiety among primary care physicians', *Soc. Sci. Med.*, 42(7):1069–75.

Yellowlees, P. M., Haynes, S., Potts, N. and Ruffin, R. E. (1988) 'Psychiatric morbidity in patients with life-threatening asthma: initial report of a controlled study', *Medical Journal of Australia*, 149(6): 246–249.

Yen, I. H., Michael, Y. L. and Perdue, L. (2009) 'Neighborhood environment in studies of health of older adults: a systematic review', *American Journal of Preventive Medicine*, 37(5): 455–463.

Zielinski, D. S. (2009) 'Child maltreatment and adult socio-economic well-being', *Child Abuse and Neglect*, 33: 666–678.

Index